Fundamental of Nursing for GNM (1st Year)

Fundamental of Nursing for GNM (1st Year)

Solved Papers with Important Theory (2016–2005)

As per INC Syllabus

Third Edition

Most Authentic and Updated Solved Question Papers

Poonam Sharda
Post Basic BSc Nursing
Baba Farid University of Health Sciences
Faridkot, Punjab, India

JAYPEE

JAYPEE BROTHERS MEDICAL PUBLISHERS

The Health Sciences Publisher

New Delhi | London

Jaypee Brothers Medical Publishers (P) Ltd

Headquarters
EMCA House
23/23-B, Ansari Road, Daryaganj
New Delhi - 110 002, India
Landline: +91-11-23272143, +91-11-23272703
+91-11-23282021, +91-11-23245672
E-mail: jaypee@jaypeebrothers.com

Corporate Office
4838/24, Ansari Road, Daryaganj
New Delhi - 110 002, India
Phone: +91-11-43574357
Fax: +91-11-43574314
E-mail: jaypee@jaypeebrothers.com

Overseas Office
J.P. Medical Ltd
83 Victoria Street, London
SW1H 0HW (UK)
Phone: +44 20 3170 8910
E-mail: info@jpmedpub.com

EU GPSR Authorised Representative
Logos Europe, 9 rue Nicolas Poussin
17000, La Rochelle, France
Phone: +33 (0) 6 67 93 73 78
E-mail: contact@logoseurope.eu

Website: www.jaypeebrothers.com
Website: www.jaypeedigital.com

Fundamental of Nursing for GNM (1st Year)

First Edition: 2013

Second Edition: 2014

Third Edition: 2017, Reprint: **2026**

ISBN: 978-93-5270-082-0

Printed at: Samrat Offset Pvt. Ltd.

Dedicated to

My Parents

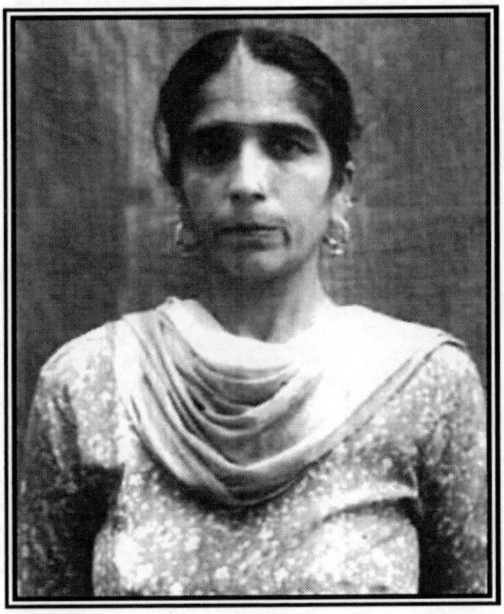

Smt Raj Rani

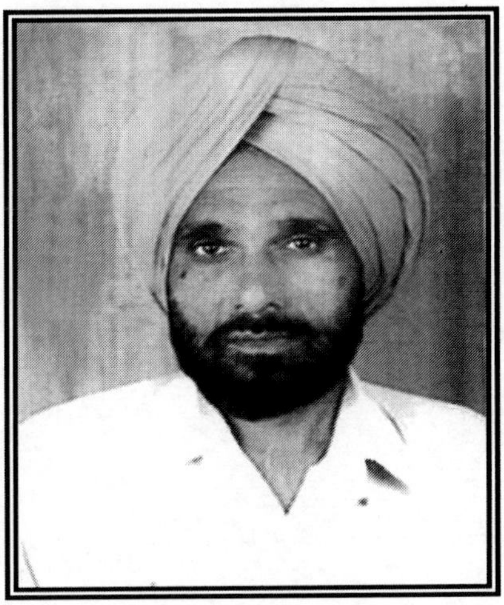

Sh Rajkumar

Preface

It is matter of great pride to present Nursing Solved Question Papers for the first year students of General Nursing and Midwifery (GNM).

As a student, I found difficulty in getting an authentic question bank during my exams. However, there were few books available in the market but they were not having the authentic questions with relevant answers so, I have compiled this question bank which appeared in Baba Farid University of Punjab as per INC regulations.

Fundamental of Nursing for GNM is written with great attention and concentration keeping in mind the basic requirements of Ist year nursing students. It contains solved question papers of Fundamental of Nursing with detailed explanations and important theory given at the beginning of every subject.

I am sure that this book will prove really beneficial to nursing students and will enable them to prepare well for their examination even without books.

Poonam Sharda

Acknowledgments

I am thankful to the God who strengthens me in each and every second in all my work by showing His blessings abundantly through various resources which helped me in accomplishment of the entire task in my life.

My sincere heartfelt thanks to my respected parents Sh Rajkumar and Smt Raj Rani for their help, support and encouragement given to me to achieve this level. Without their help this would not have been possible for me to complete this project.

My sincere thanks goes to Jaypee Brothers Medical Publishers for giving me great opportunity to publish this book.

INC Syllabus

FUNDAMENTALS OF NURSING

Hours: 174

COURSE DESCRIPTION

This course is designed to help students develop an ability to meet the basic health need of the patients with regard to nursing care and develop skill in the competencies required for rendering effective patient care.

GENERAL OBJECTIVES

Upon completion of this course, the student will be able to:

- Describe the physical mental and social adjustment required of a sick individual and his family
- Carry-out basic nursing techniques and care with the application of sound scientific principles
- Explain the concept of comprehensive nursing care
- Develop skills in assessment, planning, implementation and evaluation of the nursing care rendered to the patients
- Communicate effectively and establish good interpersonal relationship with the patients, their relatives and other health team members
- Demonstrate skills in observation, recording and reporting
- Recognize and utilize opportunities for planning and implementing need based health teaching programme(s) for individuals, groups, families and communities.

COURSE CONTENT

Unit I: Introduction to Nursing

- **Nursing:** Definition, meaning, nature, scope, principles and history of nursing
- **Nurse:** Definition and meaning, preparation of a nurse qualities-personal, professional
- Ethics in nursing, role and responsibilities of a nurse

- **Health care agencies:** Hospital and community, types of hospitals and their functions
- Holistic approach to nursing
- Comprehensive nursing care.

Unit II: Nursing Care of the Patient/Client

- Introduction to the sick and well
- Determinants of health status
- **Patient/Client:** As an individual, member of the family, society, effects of illness and hospitalization on patient and his family
- **Admission of a patient:** Patient unit, set-up and care admission procedure, reception of patient, care of patient belongings.

Bed and Bed Making

- Principle of bed-making, factor to be considered in selecting and making bed, different types of beds and their uses.

Maintenance of Therapeutic Environment

Temperature, light, noise and humidity.

Psychosocial Environment

Meaning and its importance, aesthetic consideration in the environment, colour scheme beauty and flower arrangements.

Nursing Process and Nursing Care Plan

Meaning importance and steps in development.

Recording and Reporting

Importance, types and nurses responsibilities.

Discharging a Patient

- Preparation of the patient physically and mentally, discharge procedure, hospital policies, preparation of the patients relatives for discharge
- Follow-up and rehabilitation revisit, treatment compliance and referral.

Unit III: Basic Nursing Care and Needs of the Patient

Hygienic Needs and Physical Needs

- Importance of maintaining good personal and environmental hygiene in health and disease

- Nurse role in maintaining good personal and environmental hygiene
- Care of skin and mucous membrane
- Bed bath, care of hair, eyes, nose, ears, teeth, genitalia, hands and feet.

Nutritional Needs

- Importance of diet in health and disease, factors affecting the normal nutrition in sickness, nurse role in maintaining good nutrition, feeding helpless patients, maintenance of intake and output record.

Elimination Needs

- **Problem in sickness:** Constipation and diarrhea, retention and incontinence of urine
- Nurse role in meeting elimination needs.

Safety Needs

- Environmental hazards, role of nurses in prevention of health hazards
- Interpersonal relationship, cultural/spiritual/religious needs.

Activity and Exercises

Importance of activity and exercise in health and sickness, active and passive exercise.

Physical Comforts

Comfort: Meaning and its importance in health and disease, factors promoting and inhibiting physical comfort, comfort devices and their uses, body mechanics, positions.

Moving, Shifting and Lifting of Patient

- **Care of pressure points, bedsores:** Causes, signs, symptoms, prevention and nursing care
- Shifting of patient from one side to another, from bed to wheelchair and bed to stretcher.

Unit IV: Assessment of Patient/Client

Principles and importance of assessment, methods of assessment: Observation, palpation, auscultation, percussion, developing skill in observation.

Physical Assessment

Height, weight, posture, speech.

Physiological Assessment

- Temperature, pulse, respiration and blood pressure
- Characteristics of normal and abnormal (TPR and BP) and factors influencing the variations
- Urine, stool, vomit, sputum, normal and abnormal behaviour and its deviation.

Unit V: Therapeutic Nursing Care and Procedures Asepsis

- Handwashing, hand scrubbing, use of mask, gown, gloves
- Disinfection techniques, sterilization techniques
- Autoclaving, boiling, flaming, ultraviolet rays.

Care and Sterilization

- Linen, bed, mattress, floor, walls, cupboard and other articles
- Rubber goods, dressings, instruments, needles, syringes enamel articles
- Barrier nursing and isolation.

Care of Respiratory System

- **Inhalation:** Dry inhalation, moist inhalation, jug, nelson inhaler, steam tent, electric inhalers, suction oronasal
- Collection of specimen of sputum for examination

Care of Gastrointestinal Tract

- **Preparation and giving of enema:** Retention enema, evacuation enema, suppository, passing of flatus tube.

Care of Genitourinary System

- Perineal care of terminally ill patient and patient with urinary catheter
- Collection of specimens of urine and stool for routine and cultural examination.

Care of Skin and Mucous Membranes

- **Cold application:** Ice cap, cold packs, use of evaporating lotion
- **Hot application:** Use of hot water bottle, dry fomentation, moist fomentation, medicated fomentation.

Unit VI: Basic Needs and Care in Special Conditions

- Care of patient with fever, unconscious patient, patient with fluid imbalance, patient with dyspnoea
- Care of terminally ill patient
- Care of physically handicapped.

Dying patient

- Signs and symptoms of approaching death, needs of the dying patient and his relatives, care of the dying, last offices, packing of dead bodies in noncommunicable and communicable diseases.

Unit VII: Introduction to Pharmacology

- Concept of pharmacology
- Classification of drugs
- Administration of drugs
- General action of drugs
- Nursing implications in administration of drugs.

First Aid

Hours: 20

COURSE DESCRIPTION

This course is designed to help students develop and understanding of community emergencies and be able to render first aid services as and when need arises.

General Objectives

Upon completion of this course, the students will be able to:

- Describe the rules of first aid
- Demonstrate skill in rendering first aid in case of emergencies.

COURSE CONTENT

Unit I: Introduction

- Importance of first aid and rules of first aid
- Concept of emergency.

Unit II: First Aid in Emergency Situations

- Fire, burns, fractures, accidents, poisoning, drowning, haemorrhages, insect bites, foreign bodies
- Transportation of the injured
- Bandaging and splinting.

Unit III: Community Emergencies and Resource Community Emergencies

- Fire, explosions, floods, earthquakes, famines
- Immediate and late role of nurses
- Need for rehabilitation

Community Resources

- Police Assistance
- **Voluntary agencies:** Local, national and international agencies
- **Ambulance services:** Their functions in relation to emergencies.

PERSONAL HYGIENE

Hours: 20

COURSE DESCRIPTION

This course is designed to help students acquire the concept of health, an understanding of the principles of personal health and its relation to nursing in health and disease.

GENERAL OBJECTIVES

Upon completion of this course, the students will be able to:

- Explain the concept of health and hygiene
- Enumerate the principles of personal health
- Demonstrate skills to apply these principles in effective nursing care of the patients/clients as well as in her own healthy living.

COURSE CONTENT

Unit I: Introduction

Concept of health and its relation to successful living.

Unit II: Maintenance of Health

Determinants of health, building of good health habits, immunization, correction of defects, maintenance of health records.

Unit III: Physical Health

Care of skin, hair, teeth, eyes, ears, hand and feet, rest and sleep, exercise, activity, recreation, posture, nutrition, elimination, menstrual hygiene.

Unit IV: Mental Health

- Characteristics of mentally healthy person
- Mental hygiene in intrauterine, infancy, childhood, adolescence, adulthood and old age.

Contents

Important Theory

1. Principles applied to the nursing procedures.

NURSING PRINCIPLES

- **Safety:** It means prevention of mechanical, thermal, chemical and bacteriological injuries to the patient and the workers and protection from all nuisance.
- **Therapeutic effectiveness:** It is to achieve the purpose for which a procedure is done.
- **Comfort:** To provide comfort to give satisfaction to the patient and the workers.
- **Use of resources:** It implies the right use and the economy, time, energy and material.
- **Good workmanship:** It is the art of doing.
- **Individuality:** It is to consider the needs and problems of particular patient when a procedure is done.
- **Scientific principles:** It is the application of medical biological, physical and social sciences:
  - Anatomy and physiology
  - Pharmacology
  - Psychology
  - Microbiology
  - Physics
  - Sociology
  - Nutrition
  - Chemistry.

2. Prevention of cross-infection in the hospital.

Ans.
- The hospital should be well ventilated.
- Maintain the general cleanliness of the hospital.
- Sweeping and mopping of the floor should be done daily with antiseptic lotions.
- All articles kept clean and dry.

- Once a weak roof is swept to remove the beds, lockers, stools, etc.
- The mattress, pillow and other unwashed articles are exposed to sunlight and aired.
- Periodical whitewashing of the walls, painting of the doors and windows, etc.
- Safe food and water supply: Many diseases are transmitted through food and water kitchen and pantry are protected from flies.
- Safe disposal of excreta: Urine, stool, sputum, etc. should be disposed safely. The bedpans, urinals, sputum, etc. should be cleaned and disinfected before it is used for the next patient.
- Safe disposal of refuse: Discarded dressings, garbage, etc. collected daily and burnt to prevent the spread of infection.
- Destruction of rodents and insects: Rodents and insects play great role in the spread of disease, so they should be destroyed.

3. Nurses responsibility in moving patients.

Ans.
- Check the diagnosis and the specific precautions regarding the movement of the patient.
- Check the level of consciousness and the ability to follow instruction.
- Check the ability for self-care.
- Abilities and limitation such as paralysis, fractures, splints, etc.
- Presence of muscle, skin and bone lesions and attachment, e.g. catheters and IV connections.
- The number of personnel required and available to move the patient safely.
- Articles available in the patient's unit such as a stretcher, IV, poles, clamps for disconnecting tubes, holder for drainage bags, etc.

PREPARATION OF THE PATIENT AND THE UNIT

- Provide privacy and avoid draughts.
- Explain the procedure to the patient and tell him how it helps you.
- Adjust the bed to the working height lower the side rails, lock the wheels of the bed.
- Change wet or soiled linen.
- Offer the bedpan if needed.
- Remove all comfort devices used for patient.
- Clamp catheter and nasogastric tube, other tube if any.
- Attach IV pole to stretcher.
- Position the foot stool, if needed.

AFTER CARE

- Make sure that the patient is comfortable.
- Replace the pillow and other comfort devices as needed.
- Assess the patient for pain or discomfort.
- Tidy up the unit.
- Chart in the nurses record.

4. Purpose of bed making

Ans.
- To provide the patient with a safe and comfortable bed to take rest and sleep.
- To give to the unit or ward a neat appearance.
- To adapt to the needs of the patient and to be ready for any emergency or critical condition of illness.
- To economies time, material and effort.
- To prevent bedsore.
- To promote cleanliness.
- To establish an effective nurse-patient relationship.
- To provide active and passive exercise to the patients.
- To help the relatives to learn to care for sick at home.

5. Objectives of operation bed.

Ans.
- To make a bed that will be comfortable and safe for the patient who is recovering from anesthesia.
- To be prepared to meet any emergency.
- To provide warmth.
- To protect the mattresses and pillows and facilitate remaking the parts as necessary.
- For the quick transfer of the patient from the trolley to the bed and to care for the patient without loss of time.

6. Purpose of blanket bed.

Ans.
- To carry the weight of the bed clothes off from the painful joints.
- To keep the patient warm.
- To promote elimination through the skin.

7. Importance of observation in nursing.

Ans.
- It is a chance to learn to know the patient and to understand the condition of his physical, mental and spiritual well-being.
- Through observation, any changes in the condition of the patient, improvement or regression, may be detected.
- Accurate observation helps the physician to make a correct diagnosis and to prescribe treatments.
- It helps to determine the cause and extent of disease.

- It helps the nurse to plan the nursing care in such a way, that it will produce maximum benefit and comfort to the patient.
- Data obtained by observation might be the deciding factor between life and death.
- Correct observation saves the life of the patient in the critical condition of illness.
- Accurate observation helps to prevent complications in the patient by detecting the early signs of complication.
- It helps the nurse to use the safety measures to prevent accidents.
- It safeguards the patient and his family by noting the early sign in case of communicable disease.
- It contributes to one's own learning as well as it promotes research studies.
- Observation is the basis of all scientific works and all intelligent and effective action.
- A hospital is able to analyze the quality of its services through carefully recorded observations.

8. Nurses responsibilities in the collection of specimens.

PREPARATION OF THE PATIENT

Explain the procedure to the patient, what specimen to collect, when to collect, how to collect and the amount to be collected. Provide appropriate container and demonstrate to him how to use it. Ask the patient to wash the external genitalia area with soap and water and then rinse it with water alone before collection the urine specimen.

Preparation of the Equipment

- All specimen collect in clean and dry containers.
- Use wide mouth container.
- Sterilize container used for culture specimen.
- Wax like lined disposable cups are used for the collection and stool specimens.
- Large container used for 24 hours specimen.
- Clean slides are used for smears.

9. Purpose of bed bath.

Ans.
- To clean the body of dirt and bacteria.
- To increase elimination through the skin.
- To prevent bedsores.
- To stimulate circulation.

- To induce sleep.
- To provide comfort to the patient.
- To relieve fatigue.
- To give the patient a sense of well-being.
- To regulate body temperature.
- To provide active and passive exercise.
- To observe objective symptoms.
- To give the nurse an opportunity for health teaching.
- To establish an effective nurses health patient relationship.

10. Prevention of pediculosis.

Ans. Prevention is easier than controlling. Personal hygiene plays important role like combing the hair daily, washing it frequently keep the skin and clothing clean will solve the problem. Any patient complaining of itching the head, needs though examination of the hair and sleep, body and linen to discover lice.

PARASITICIDES USED IN TREATMENT

- DDT 5% or 10%.
- Carbolic lotion 1%.
- Equal part of kerosene oil and coconut oil.
- Preparations containing gamma benzene hexachloride available in the market.

APPLICATION OF PARASITICIDE

It applied is thoroughly on the scalp and left for overnight, on the next day bath is given and the linen is changed. The linen should be thoroughly disinfected to remove the lice from the clothes. Parasiticides are not effective against the nits (egg) the procedure is repeated after a week.

11. Modification of nutrients in therapeutic diet.

Ans. a. **Carbohydrate:** Carbohydrates are well-tolerated and are necessary to maintain the stores of liver glycogen. It is important for a patient with high fever, liver disease, hyperthyroidism, etc. In absence of carbohydrates the body fat may be used for energy which may result in the formation of ketone bodies and accumulate in the body is called ketosis.

b. **Fat:** Fats are not tolerated in illness especially if nausea and vomiting are present. Adequate amount of carbohydrate can replace the requirement of body fat.

c. **Protein:** When there is infection, the protein metabolism is usually increased because of the increases destruction of protein. If adequate amount of protein is not given the patient will lose weight. In kidney and liver damages, the protein intake should be high.

d. **Minerals:** Minerals should be maintained in illness especially calcium and iron. In hypertension sodium and potassium may be restricted.

e. **Vitamins:** Fat soluble vitamin added in diet if the patient on fat restricted diet. Vitamin C increases in fever and for wound healing.

f. **Fluid:** It is important to prevent dehydration especially when fluid is lost from the body in excess amount. In severe cases, IV fluid given, fluids with protein necessary for patient who are on liquid diets for a long time.

12. Purpose of Fowler's position.

Ans.
- To drainage of the abdominal cavity is desired.
- To localize infection, e.g. peritonitis.
- To relieve breathing difficulty.
- To relieve tension on the abdominal sutures.
- To relax the large muscle of the back and thighs.
- To give the patient a sense of well-being and make it easier for him for self-care.

13. Purpose of cardiac position.

Ans.
- To give comfortable position for patient with cardiac asthma.
- Used for cardiac disease patient.
- To relieve fatigue.
- To prevent embolism.

14. Prevention and treatment of retention of urine.

Ans. Before catheterization, an intelligent nurse will use all her knowledge and skill to aid the patient to empty the bladder by natural means. Methods used in inducing urination are:

- Assist the patient to his or her normal position. For voiding male patient may find it easier to void when standing rather than sitting position.
- A female patient may find it easier to void using a commode at the side of the bed rather than using bedpan on the bed.
- Provide privacy even children because no body able to void in front of others.

- Offer a bedpan or urinal that is warm. A bedpan that is cold to touch may cause contraction of the perineal muscles.
- Local application of heat to the perineum and lower abdominal muscle.
- Running water within the hearing of the patient stimulates micturition.
- Provide enough time for micturition never show hurry.
- Reassure the patient by psychological support.
- A hot enema. If permitted, may relieve the retention of the urine.
- Give fluids freely unless contraindicated.

  Some diuretics such as lemon drinks, weak tea, coffee, etc. are given in plenty to induce urination when all these nursing measures are falling, catheterization of the bladder is done with the doctors, permission.

15. Purpose of fomentations.

Ans.
- To relieve pain and congestion.
- To relieve inflammation.
- To relieve retention of urine.
- To promote suppuration.
- To stimulate peristalsis and to relieve tympanitis.
- To relieve intestinal and renal colic.
- To soften the crust and for the easy removal of a crust.
- To relieve muscular spasm.
- To relieve congestion in the internal organs.

16. Safety measure of drug administration.

Ans. The "Five Right" ensures safety in giving drugs:
- Right patient.
- Right drug.
- Right dose.
- Right time.
- Right method.

17. Ethical and legal aspects regarding medication.

Ans.
- Under the law nurses are responsible for their own actions regardless of a written order. It is expected to know for all nurses the minimum and maximum dose of every medicine that she administers. If a nurse gives an injection of pethedine 200 mg to a patient instead of 50 mg the nurse is responsible for harm that has taken place in the patient.

- The nurse should know the law about the use of narcotics. The narcotics should be kept under the safe custody of nurses and account should be maintained for the administration of these drugs.

The following information should be recorded when narcotics are given:

- Name of patient
- Name of drug
- Dosage
- Date
- Time.

Signature of person who prepared and gave the narcotic and name of doctor who ordered the drug:

- The nurse responsibility includes prevention of medication errors by observing the fine rights of giving medications.
- Observing side effect and recording is responsibility of nurse.
- Another legal responsibility of the nurse is when she is involved in the experimental drug program.

18. Factors affecting appetite.

Ans. The appetite is increased by:

- Sight and smell of food.
- Food preference.
- Physical and mental relaxation.
- Regularity in eating.
- Pleasant environment.
- Exercise.

The appetite is decreased by:

- Physical and mental fatigue.
- Hurry, worry and fear.
- Unpleasant environment and experiences.
- Lack of exercise.
- Irregular meals.
- Long spacing of meal timings.

19. Classification of Hospitals.

Ans. Hospitals are classified according to the size or bed capacity, ownership or control, purpose or clinical facilities:

Size or Bed Capacity

The size of an institution is determined by the number of beds it has. A bed capacity of 100 or less is considered as small hospital. The bed capacity of

100 to 300 is considered to be medium sized hospital and a bed capacity of 300 to 1000 is considered as a large hospital.

Ownership or Control

According to the ownership or control, it can be classified into governmental or nongovernmental. Hospital controlled by government agencies are tax supplied. Nongovernment institutions are supported by patient's fees, gifts and endowments, etc.

Nongovernment hospital are further classified as other proprietary or nonprofit organization. Nonprofit hospitals are called charitable hospital.

Purpose or Clinical Facilities

The hospitals are classified into general hospitals and special hospitals according to the type of service they offer. A general hospital has various clinical services available to patients such as medical, surgical, pediatric psychiatric, tuberculosis, etc. A special hospital limits its services to patients with a particular disease or conditions, e.g. TB (Maternity and pediatric hospitals), etc.

20. Define the following:

BANDAGING

It is a process of covering the wound or injured part.

PROPHYLACTIC

It is a measure taken to prevent a disease.

MELENA

It refers to stools that are very dark or black because of the presence of blood.

COMPLICATION

A new disease occurs due to old disease as not treated.

SPECIFIC GRAVITY

Specific gravity is the ratio of the density of a substance to the density of another substance accepted as a standard.

CAPILLARY ACTION

Capillary action is defined as the rise or fall of a liquid in a tube of fine bare.

LAW OF BUOYANCY

The low of buoyancy states that a body immersed in a fluid (a gas or a liquid sustained) up by a force equal to the weight of the fluid it displaces.

RADIOACTIVE ISOTOPES

Those forms of element in which the nucleus is instable and which exhibit radioactivity are known as radioactive isotopes.

ISOTONIC SOLUTION

It an aqueous solution on each side of a membrane, has equal concentration and some osmotic pressure. It is called isotonic solution.

BUFFERS

Certain molecules and ions which maintain the constancy of hydrogen ion concentrations in a liquid are called buffers.

STOMATITIS

Inflammation of the mucous membrane of the mouth.

HALITOSIS

It is the comprehensive nursing care provided to the patient through nursing process.

FIRST AID

First aid is the immediate treatment given to the victim of trauma or sudden illness before medical help is made available.

POISONING

A poison is a substance which when taken into the body in sufficient quantity will harm or destroy life.

WOUND

A wound is a breach in the continuity of the skin as a result of injury.

FRACTURE

A fracture is a breach in the continuity of a bone due to direct trauma force of contraction of powerful muscles.

HYPOXIA

It is a condition in which the lungs do not get sufficient air or oxygen.

DISLOCATION

It is disruption of a joint, so that the bones forming the joint move away from each other.

FIGURE OF EIGHT

The bandage is applied obliquely up and down alternately, so that the loops appear like the figure of eight.

T BANDAGE

It can be made from two strips of gauze or bandage. Folding one at right angles over the middle of the other.

21. First aid of fracture.

Ans. Aims of Management:

- To control hemorrhage
- To reduce pain
- To prevent further damage
- To make patient comfortable
- To get medical aid at the earliest:
  - Fracture often occurs in major accidents. Therefore, it is common to find other injuries also. The first must decide which is more urgent and should be treated first.
  - There may be more than one fracture in the same patient or even in the same limb.
  - If there is no immediate danger of life, temporary attention to fracture is enough.
  - Treat the fracture on the spot, so that the fracture ends are established and patient is ready for transport handle very gently, all necessary movement of the injured part.
  - Send for medical aid or send the patient to hospital as quickly as possible also inform patient relatives. Treat for shock.

- If the broken ends of the bone show out, do not wash the wound or apply antiseptics to the ends of the bone.
- Do not handle the fracture unnecessarily.
- Never attempt to bring the bones to normal position or reduce the fracture.

22. First aid management of head injury.

Ans.
- Give comfortable position to the patient.
- Reassure the patient and family.
- Open head wounds should be covered and pressure applied to control bleeding unless there appears to be underlying depressed or compound skull fracture.
- Do not attempt to remove foreign or any penetrating objects from the wound.
- Patient may die due to insufficient respiration and poor brain O_2 so give artificial respiration at that spot by mouth to mouth respiration method.
- Nothing should be given to the patient through mouth in case of several head injuries.
- Elevate the head end side of the patient, so that the patient may not aspirate the secretion.
- Clean the mouth of the patient with clean cloth.
- Shift the patient to the hospital as soon as possible.
- In hospital, start oxygen to the patient.
- Start IV fluids to maintain the tissue perfusion.

23. Prevention of poisoning.

Ans. Cure can be available nowadays for every thing but it is better if these kind of problems can be prevented as prevention is always better than cure:

- The storage and handling of poisonous substance should be done carefully.
- Label all the poisonous substance and teach children not to touch the containers.
- Do not place the container of any poisonous substance along with other containers in kitchen.
- All the chemicals of any medicines should be kept away from the reach of children.
- While giving any medicines to children supervise him.
- No medicines should be taken without the prescription by doctor or some medical professional.

- Do not let infants and children play where the poisonous substances are kept.
- Do not put poisons in containers of any food material.
- While spraying any poisonous substance, do not accompany and children along with you.
- DDT like substance should not be put on floor of a room where children play.
- Wash your hands properly after working with any poisonous substance.
- Education to high-risk group or attendants as parents are educated for prevention of accidental poisoning in children.

24. First aid management of drowing.

Ans.
- Quickly remove any obstruction such as seaweed from the casualty mouth and begin artificial ventilation immediately.
- If he is still in the water, it may be possible to begin ventilation there.
- If within your depth use one arm to support the casualty to support his head and seal his nose. While you perform mouth to mouth ventilation if in deeper water give the occasional breath of air, etc. while towing the casualty ashore.
- When you can place him on a firm surface, check breathing pulse and continue resuscitation, if necessary.
- As soon as possible casualty begins breathing, place in the recovery position.
- Keep him warm, if possible, remove wet clothing and dry him off cover with spare clothes, or towels.
- Do no allow him to sit-up.
- Remove false teeth if present.
- Pull tongue forward.
- Do not attempt to force water out or stomach.
- Raise the middle part of the body with your hands around the belly.
- During artificial respiration as helpers to call for doctor and ambulance.
- The casualty should always receive medical attention even if he appears to recover rapidly.

Fundamental of Nursing
November 2016

Time: 3 Hours **Maximum Marks: 75**

Note: *Attempt all the questions. Attempt all parts of question at same place.*

1. **(a) Define the following terms:**
   i. Nursing
   ii. Health
   iii. Hospital acquired infection
   iv. Respiration
   v. Gingivitis

   (b) Enlist the qualities of a nurse
   (c) Discuss the various methods of physical exams. (5 + 5 + 5 = 15)

2. **(a) Define sterilization and enlist the various methods of sterilization.**
   (b) Which is the best method of sterilization?
   (c) Explain about the barrier in nursing care. (5 + 5 + 5 = 15)

3. **Write the Nursing responsibilities of the following:**
   (a) Collection of 24 hours urine.
   (b) While giving bed bath.
   (c) Oxygen inhalation. **(5 + 5 + 5 = 15)**

4. **(a) Discuss the importance of documentation in nursing.**
   (b) Enlist the principles to maintain records and reports.
   (c) Write about the various types of records to be maintained in hospitals. (5 + 5 + 5 = 15)

5. **Write short note of the following:**
   (a) Comfort devices or body mechanics
   (b) Handwashing or restraining
   (c) Urine analysis or oral medication (5 + 5 + 5 = 15)

SOLVED QUESTION PAPER NOVEMBER 2016

1. (a) Define the following terms: **(5 + 5 + 5 = 15)**
   i. Nursing
   ii. Health
   iii. Hospital acquired infection
   iv. Respiration
   v. Gingivitis

(b) Enlist the qualities of a nurse

(c) Discuss the various methods of physical exams. **(5 + 5 + 5 = 15)**

NURSING

Nursing is a dynamic, therapeutic and educative process in meeting the health needs of the individual, family and society.

HEALTH

It is defined as 'state of complete physical, mental, social and spiritual well-being, not merely an absence of disease or infirmity'.

HOSPITAL ACQUIRED INFECTION

A client develops an infection that was not present or was incubating at the time of admission to the health care setting.

RESPIRATION

It is the act of breathing. It is the process of taking in oxygen and giving out carbon dioxide. Respiration constitutes inspiration, expiration and a pause.

GINGIVITIS

It is an inflammation of the gums.

QUALITIES OF A NURSE

Refer paper 2008 question no 1(b)

VARIOUS METHODS OF PHYSICAL EXAMS

There are four methods for physical exam:

Inspection

It is the systematic visual examination of the clients. It involves observation of the color, shape, size, symmetry, position and movements. It also uses the sense of smell to detect odor and sense of hearing to detect sounds.

General inspection of a client focuses on the following areas:

- Overall appearance of health or illness
- Signs of distress
- Facial expression and mood
- Body size
- Grooming and personal hygiene

Palpation

It is use of the hands and fingers to gather information through touch. It is the assessment technique, which uses sense of touch.

The hands and fingers are sensitive tools and can assess temperature, turgor, texture, moisture, vibrations, size, position, consistency, masses and fluid. The dorsum (back) of hand and fingers used to measure temperature. Vibration is palpated best with the palm of the hand.

The nurse's hands should be warm and fingernails short and the touch should be gentle and respectful.

Percussion

It is the examination by tapping the fingers on the body to determine the condition of the internal organs by the sounds that are produced.

Percussion provides information about the nature of an underlying structure. It is used to outline the size of an organ such as bladder or liver. There are two types of percussion, direct and indirect. Direct percussion is accomplished by tapping an area directly with the finger tip of the middle finger or thumb.

Auscultation

It is the process of listening the sounds that are generated within the body. Auscultation is usually done with the help of a stethoscope, when auscultating a part, that area should be exposed and should be quiet:

1. Pitch (ranging from high to low)
2. Loudness (ranging from soft to loud)
3. Quality (gurgling or swishing)
4. Duration (short, medium and long).

2. (a) Define sterilization and enlist the various methods of sterilization.

(b) Which is the best method of sterilization?

(c) Explain about the barrier in nursing care.

STERILIZATION AND ITS METHODS

Sterilization

It is the process by which an object becomes free of all the microorganisms including the spores.

Methods of Sterilization

Boiling

Total immersion in boiling water at 100 °C for 10 minutes. It is a common or reliable method of disinfecting instruments.

Disinfection by Disinfectants

A chemical disinfectant acts by coagulating the bacteria protein or by changing the composition of protein so that no longer exists in the same form. It is also called as cold sterilization.

Fumigation

Total surface exposure to formaldehyde gas under conditions of control humidity, temperature and time exposure will destroy all vegetative forms of bacteria, viruses and most of the spores. It is also known as gas sterilization.

Ultraviolet Rays Sterilization

It is effective for disinfecting working surfaces and air inside the rooms.

Steam Under Pressure or Autocalving

It is effective, widely used, economical, one of the most effective method of destroying microorganisms. This method uses high-temperature pressure, humidity to destroy bacteria life. In an autoclave, steam is present under pressure to maintain the necessary high temperature for sterilization and it allows rapid penetration of articles packed in it.

BEST METHOD OF STERILIZATION

Autoclaving or Steam Under Pressure

This method is most commonly and widely used to destroy microorganism. In autoclaving, the steam should be at 15 lbs to 20 lbs/inch^2 pressure at 121 °C temperature for 30 minutes. This method is generally employed for surgical linens, gloves, gauze, cotton, etc.

BARRIER IN NURSING CARE

Barrier nursing or isolation technique is intended to confine the micro-organism within a given and recognized area. There are a number of isolation techniques and precautions used to prevent the spread of infection.

Respiratory Isolation

It is used when pathogens are spread on droplets from the respiratory tract. In this type of isolation, masks are generally worn by the nurses. Gowns are also worn when caring for the small infants because of the possibility of drooling by the infants. The nurse suffering from respiratory diseases should not attend to the client.

Enteric Isolation

Enteric isolation is indicated when the pathogens are transmitted in feces. For this type of isolation it is not necessary to wear a mask, but it is recommended that gloves and gowns should be worn while handling soiled articles.

The soiled articles such as linen should be disinfected before it is sent to washerman.

Wound and Skin Isolation

This type of isolation is for pathogens which are found in wounds and can be transmitted by the contact with the wounds. Strict isolation should be used while caring for client with abscesses, boils, infected burns, gas gangrene, rabies, tetanus, venereal disease, scabies, etc.

Blood Isolation

It is used to prevent transmission of pathogens that are found in the blood. Any equipment infected with blood should be carefully disinfected to prevent this type of infection.

Face Masks

Masks are generally used to prevent the spread of microorganisms to and from the client through the respiratory tract. Masks should be worn only once and then discarded to ensure effective filtering of microorganism. Masks should not be worn outside the unit. Masks need to cover both mouth and nose and fit snugly around the face to prevent the escape of microorganism around the sides.

Gloves

Gloves are used in the medical asepsis to protect the nurse from pathogens. Gloves used for this purpose are clean but need not be sterile. Gloves must be changed between the two activities.

3. Write the Nursing responsibilities of the following:

(a) Collection of 24 hours urine.
(b) While giving bed bath.
(c) Oxygen inhalation.

COLLECTION OF URINE SPECIMEN

Refer important theory question no 8

NURSING RESPONSIBILITY WHILE GIVING BED BATH

Preliminary Assessment

- Check the physician orders to see the specific precautions if any.
- Asses the clients need for bathing.
- Assess client ability for self-care.
- Assess cardiorespiratory functioning.
- Check TPR and BP.
- Assess clients mental ability to follow directions.
- Check the clients preference for soap, powder, etc.
- Check all articles available in client unit or not.

Preparation of Articles

All needed equipment should be at hand and conveniently placed before beginning the procedure so as to avoid leaving the client unnecessarily until the entire procedure has been completed. Arrange articles in the order of use.

Preparation of the Client and Unit

- Explain the sequence of the procedure to the client and explain how the client can assist you
- Move the unnecessary items from the work area
- Place the articles needed conveniently on the bedside table.
- Adjust the height of the bed to the comfortable working of the nurse.
- Bring the client to the edge of the bed and towards the nurse to prevent overreaching
- Check the room temperature and warm it if necessary
- Close the windows if necessary and put off the fan to prevent draughts
- Provide privacy by the means of curtains.
- Remove the top bed linen or fanfold them to the foot end of the bed, leaving a sheet or bath blanked over the client
- Offer bedpan or urinal if necessary
- Keep the client flat if the condition permits. Remove extra pillows and bact rest
- Remove the personal clothing and cover the client with the bath blanket.

After Care of the Client and Articles

- Replace the clients personal clothing
- Straighten the bed linen
- Remove the bath blanket and put it for washing
- Change the bed linen if needed
- Offer a hot drink if permitted.
- Cut short the finger nails and the toe nails
- Comb the hair and arrange the hair
- Position the client for comfort and proper alignment.

- Take all articles to the utility room.
- Disinfect the bath basin and the wash clothes.
- Send soiled linen into the laundry
- Wash hands
- Take opportunity to teach the client or his relatives about the personal hygiene.

OXYGEN INHALATION

- Check the proper O_2 cylinder or pipeline, no blockage in the catheter or no leakage to be present.
- Humidified O_2 should be given to avoid burning of mucous membrane.
- Give intermittent O_2 and not the continuous and as advised by the doctor.
- Check the improvement has taken place after O_2 administration or not.
- Do not use flaming items as match box, rubber toys or do not smoke at that area.
- Check the apparatus daily in order to meet in an emergency or its functioning conditions.

4. (a) Discuss the importance of documentation in nursing.
(b) Enlist the principles to maintain records and reports.
(c) Write about the various types of records to be maintained in hospitals.

IMPORTANCE OF DOCUMENTATION

Refer paper 2008 question no 3(a)

PRINCIPLES TO MAINTAIN RECORDS

Date and Time

Document the date and time of each recording. Record the time in the conventional manner, e.g. 9 AM to 3 PM, etc.

Correct Spelling

It is essential for accuracy in recording. In cause of doubt, check the dictionary and use the correct spelling.

Appropriateness

Record only information that pertains to the clients health problems and care.

Legal Prudence

Accurate and complete documentation give legal protection to the nurse and other health care personal and the client.

Accuracy

Client's name and identification date must be written on each page of the clinical record.

Completeness

Document all information necessary to explain the events in a shift. Anyone reading the document should have a clear picture of what took place or is being described.

Conciseness

Good charting is concise and brief.

Legibility

Writing must be clear and easily readable by others.

Organization

Recording of information on the client record must follow a chronological order.

Timeliness

Documents in a timely manner can help avoid errors.

Corrections

Two types of corrections made to a record are correcting a written entry and adding an entry later when and error occurs, do not erase it.

Omissions

Blank space are not to be left on the chart.

Signature

A written signature must follow every entry into a client's record.

Confidentiality

All client's records kept confidential properly according to the policies of the agency.

VARIOUS TYPES OF RECORDS TO BE MAINTAINED IN HOSPITALS

Refer paper 2008 question no 3(b)

5. **Write short note of the following.**
   (a) Comfort devices or body mechanics
   (b) Handwashing or restraining
   (c) Urine analysis or oral medication.

COMFORT DEVICES

Refer paper 2005 question no 4(b)

BODY MECHANICS

It is defined as using alignment, posture and balance in a coordinated effort to perform activities such as lifting, bending and moving. Correct body mechanics are essential and help avoid work-related musculoskeletal injuries, diminish excessive strain and fatigue and minimize the potential for client injury.

Importance of Good Body Mechanics

- Proper body alignment and posture prevent fatigue and deformities
- Good posture promotes normal physiological functions of the body. It aids in circulation and digestion
- It helps to maintain the balance of the body without undue strain on the body parts
- It contributes to one's beauty
- Good posture prevents the development of kyphosis, lordosis, scoliosis, etc.

Principles of Body Mechanics

- Proper balancing of all body parts helps to conserve energy.
- Stability of the body is maintained by having a greater base of support.
- Injury and strain on the lower back can be avoided by performing pelvic tilt before the activity.
- Facing the direction of work will help to avoid the chances of injury.
- Moving an object on a level surface requires less effort.
- Reducing friction between the object moved and the surface on which it is moved required less energy.
- Holding an object close to the body requires less energy than holding it farther away.
- Muscle strain can be avoided by using the strong leg muscles when lifting, pushing and pulling.
- Smooth continuous movement are easier and safer than sudden, sharp or uncontrolled movements.

HANDWASHING

The infection can be transferred from person to person by contaminated hands. Careful handwashing of the hands reduces the number of bacteria. Handwashing involves both mechanical and chemical action.

Points to be Kept in Mind while Washing Hands

- Cut short nails, a long nail will give roof to the dirt and microorganism.
- Remove the jewellery of any type.
- Open the tap, wet the hands and forearm.
- Water should flow from the area of least contamination to the area of more contamination.
- Apply soap, rinse the soap before it is returned to the container.
- Wash hand thoroughly.
- Use brush to dislodge the dirt from under the nail beds.
- Rinse hands by keeping the hands well below the elbow level.
- Repeat the procedure to ensure thorough cleanliness.
- Turn off the water tap using a paper towel because the handle is contaminated.

URINE ANALYSIS

Color

Take a clean glass jar and pour urine into it and place it on a table against light, note the color, normally it is pale, yellow or amber color.

Appearance

After noting the color, inspect the whole urine for the presence of sediments of suspended articles. Normal urine is clear.

Odor

Normal urine has aromatic odor.

Reaction

To test urine reaction, normal urine is acidic in reaction.

Specific Gravity

Specific gravity of the urine is the relation of the weight of a known quantity of water.

Volume

Take a graduated jar and measure the urine.

ORAL MEDICATION

Refer paper 2008 question no 4(a)

Fundamental of Nursing
October 2015

Time: 3 Hours | **Maximum Marks: 75**

Note: *Attempt all questions. Please attempt all parts of the question in sequence.*

1. Define the following: 2×5 = 10
   (a) Dyspnea
   (b) Autoclaving
   (c) Temperature
   (d) Pulse
   (e) Bradycardia

2. (a) Define blood pressure. 2+7+6 = 15
   (b) Explain the factors affecting the blood pressure.
   (c) Write down the diet for the hypertension patient.

3. Write down the purposes of the following: 5+5+5 = 15
   (a) Mouth care
   (b) Hot application
   (c) Soap and water Enema

4. Write down nursing care of the following: 5+5+5 = 15
   (a) Bed sore
   (b) Incontinence of urine
   (c) Dehydration

5. Write short notes on any four of the following: 4×5 = 20
   (a) Hospital
   (b) Barrier Nursing
   (c) Oral Medication
   (d) Cross infection
   (e) Sterilization

SOLVED PAPER OCTOBER 2015

1. Define the following:
   (a) Dyspnea
   (b) Autoclaving
   (c) Temperature
   (d) Pulse
   (e) Bradycardia

DYSPNEA

It is defined as difficulty in breathing.

AUTOCLAVING

It is the process of sterilization of articles by steam under pressure using an apparatus called autoclave.

TEMPERATURE

It is the balance between heat loss and heat produced by the body.

PULSE

It is an alternate expansion (rise) and fall (recoil) of an artery as the wave of blood is forced through it during the contraction of the left ventricle.

BRADYCARDIA

A pulse rate below 60 per minute in an adult is referred to be bradycardia.

2. (a) Define blood pressure.
(b) Explain the factors affecting the blood pressure.
(c) Write down the diet for the hypertension patient.

BLOOD PRESSURE

Blood pressure is the force exerted by the blood against the walls of the blood vessels as it flows against the walls of the blood vessels as it flows through the normal range of BP is 120/80 mm Hg.

FACTORS AFFECTING BLOOD PRESSURE

Age: Blood pressure is lower in children than in adults
Sex: There is no difference in BP valves between boys and girls until puberty.
Body Build: BP is higher in persons with over weight than and persons of the same age with normal weight
Race: Certain races, e.g. Negroes will have higher BP reading than other races.
Climate: Pressure norms are lower in tropical climates than temperature and highest in polar climates.
Time of the day: In all persons BP is lowest in the early morning and then rises to a peak in the evening, then it declines.
Exercise: Muscular exertion will raise the BP

Pain: Severe pain may cause temporary and marked increase in the BP.
Emotions: Fear, worry, excitement and other emotional factors will raise BP to greater level.
Posture: BP is lower when lying down than sitting or standing.
Disease condition: Diseases affecting the circulatory system and kidneys may increase BP.
Drugs: The drugs such as amyl-nitrite and nitroglycerine may cause a decrease in the BP.
Hemorrhage: Hemorrhage causes a low BP.

DIET FOR HYPERTENSION PATIENT

Hypertension develops when, for some reason, there is increased resistance to the normal circulation of blood. This may be temporary as the result of exercise emotion, pregnancy or menopause, it may be permanent, associated with atherosclerosis, cardiac failure or chronic kidney disease.
Treatment: The principles of treatment are as follows:
1. Drugs as prescribed by physician
2. Low sodium-Low fat

Daily menu for high blood pressure.

Morning	Weak tea	1Cup
Break fast	Bread or cornflakes with skimmed milk	
	Fluids	1 serving
	Weak tea	1 cup
Mid morning	Fruit juice	One glass
Lunch	Rice + chapatti, cooked dal curd, fruits, skim milk	
Evening	Biscuits	2
	Fruit juice	
Dinner	As similar to lunch	

Main focus on low salt diet should be recommended.

3. Write down the purposes of the following:
(a) Mouth care
(b) Hot application
(c) Soap and water Enema

MOUTH CARE

Refer paper 2005 question no 2(b)

PURPOSE OF HOT APPLICATION

Refer important theory question no 15

PURPOSE OF SOAP AND WATER ENEMA

Refer paper 2005 question no 2(a)

4. Write down nursing care of the following:
   (a) Bed sore
   (b) Incontinence of urine
   (c) Dehydration

BED SORE

Refer paper 2007 question no 4(a)

INCONTINENCE OF URINE

- Establishing a regular voiding schedule for the client, e.g. every 2 hrs.
- Increase the physical activity. This will improve the muscle tone
- Perineal exercises increase the muscle tone. It helps in gaining voiding control.
- Arrange toilet and bedpan within the easy reach of the client.
- Medical and surgical correction of causative factor, e.g. treatment of UTI.
- Bladder training programme: The fluid intake is to be maintained between 2000 to 3000 mL per day.
- **Skin care:** The major physical problem caused by incontinence is skin irritation and maceration washing the perineal region with soap and water exposing the skin to air circulation are.
- **Blood isolation:** This type of isolation is intended to prevent transmission of pathogens that are found in the blood. Therefore, any equipment that comes in contact with the clients blood should be carefully infected before touching another object or person. Use of mosquito net are also emphasized to prevent this type of infection.
- **Condom drainage:**
  - A male client with incontinence of urine can be safely managed with a condom drainage. In condom drainage, a condom is attached to a piece of plastic drainage tube, and inserted over the penis. The tube is connected to drainage bag.
  - **Catheterization:** Urinary catheterization is done when other possible method are fail.

DEHYDRATION

Refer paper 2007 Question no 4 (d) care of patient with diarrhea

5. **Write short notes on any four of the following:**
 (a) Hospital
 (b) Barrier Nursing
 (c) Oral Medication
 (d) Cross infection
 (e) Sterilization

HOSPITAL

A hospital is an institution for the medical and nursing care of ill and injured person needing complex services with a high-risk of complications. Hospitals are organized institutions for the care of the sick, and injured.

Functions

- **Client care:** Care of sick and injured and restoration of health
- Diagnosis and treatment of the disease
- Prevention of disease, e.g. by immunization
- Promotion of health
- Rehabilitation
- Vocational training
- Medical and nursing research
- Outpatient and inpatient services.

Types of Hospital

Refer Important theory question no 19

BARRIER NURSING

Barrier nursing or isolation technique is intended to confine the microorganisms within a given and recognized area. There are a number of isolation techniques and precautions used to prevent the spread of infection.
Respiratory isolation: Respiratory isolation is indicated in situations where the pathogens are spread on droplets from the respiratory tract. In this type of isolation masks, that are generally worn by the nurses. Gown also worn when caring for the small infants. The nurses suffering from respiratory diseases should not attend to the client.
Enteric isolation: Enteric isolation is indicated when the pathogens are transmitted in feces. It is not necessary to wear mask, but it is recommended that gloves and gowns should be worn while handling soiled particles.

Wound and skin isolation: This type of isolation is for pathogens which are found in wound and can be transmitted by the contact with the wounds. Usually gown, and gloves are worn in this type of isolation. Strict isolation techniques should be followed while caring for client with abscesses, boils, infected, burns, gas-gangrene, anthrax, rabies, tetanus, scabies, etc.

ORAL MEDICATION

It is the administration of drugs by mouth for systemic effect. It may be in the form of pills, tablets, capsule and liquids.

Five Rights of Patient in Giving Drugs

1. Right patient
2. Right drug
3. Right time
4. Right dose
5. Right method

Nursing Responsibility

- Check patient identifications
- Check doctor order, date, time, route, etc.
- Check nurses record
- Check symptoms of overdosage of drugs
- Check contra-indication
- Check character of drug
- Check form of drug available
- Check conciousness of the patient and ability to follow instructions
- Check articles available in client unit.

CROSS INFECTION

Cross infection: Infection transmitted between individuals infected with different pathogenic organisms, cross infection occurs usually in the hospitals. It is the infection of a client with a disease other than that, for which he had been admitted.

Methods of Cross Infection

- **Direct contact:** The organisms can be transmitted directly from person to person through kissing, sexual contact, droplet infection and infected hands.
- **Indirect contact:** Contact with the secretions and excretions of the infected persons.

- Through fomites, e.g. instrument, utensils, etc.
- Through contaminated food and water.
- Through insects.
- Through dust.
- Through carriers.

Prevention of Cross Infection in the Hospital

- The hospital should be well-ventilated.
- Maintain the general cleanliness of the hospital sweeping and mopping of the floor should be done daily with antiseptic lotions and damp dusting should be done to keep the articles free from dust.
  - All articles are kept clean and dry once in a week, roof is swept to remove the cobwebs
  - Bed lockers, stools, etc. should be washed and cleaned, the mattress, pillows and other unwashable articles are exposed to the sunlight and dried.
  - Periodical white washing of walls, painting of the doors and windows etc. should be done.
- **Safe food and water supply:** Many diseases are transmitted through food and water kitchen, and pantry are protected from flies. There must be provision for safe water supply.

STERILIZATION

Refer previous papers.

Fundamental of Nursing September 2015

Time: 3 Hours | **Maximum Marks: 75**

Note: *Attempt all parts of questions. Attempt all parts sequence wise.*

1. Define the following: **1×10 = 10**

a. Antiseptic
b. Rigor mortis
c. Isolation
d. Temperature
e. Asepsis
f. Blood pressure
g. Ethics in nursing
h. Tachycardia
i. Bacteriostatic
j. Respiration

2. a. Discuss the importance of documentation in nursing. **5×2 = 10**
b. Write the various types of records which are used in wards.

3. a. Define enema. **2+5+8 = 15**
b. Write the classification of enema.
c. Explain the procedure of soap and water enema.

4. a. Define nursing. **2+8 = 10**
b. Elaborate the scope of nursing.

5. Write down the purposes on any three of the following: **3×5 = 15**

a. Operation bed
b. Fowler's position
c. Cold compresses
d. Air mattress

6. Write short notes on any three of the following: **3×5 = 15**

a. Qualities of nurse
b. Holistic nursing
c. Care of rubber articles
d. Admission procedure of patient in hospital
e. Comfort devices used in hospital

SOLVED PAPER SEPTEMBER 2015

1. Define the following:

a. Antiseptic
b. Rigor mortis
c. Isolation
d. Temperature
e. Asepsis
f. Blood pressure

g. Ethics in nursing
h. Tachycardia
i. Bacteriostatic
j. Respiration

ANTISEPTIC

It is process of sterilization, use chemical substance to prevent the infection or the growth of the organism is known as antiseptic.

RIGOR MORTIS

It is the stiffening of the body after death within few hours because of coagulation of muscle plasma.

ISOLATION

It is the separation of infected person to healthy person to prevent the spreading of communicable disease.

TEMPERATURE

It is the balance between heat lost and heat gained by the body.

ASEPSIS

Freedom from infection or prevention of contact with microorganism.

BLOOD PRESSURE

Blood pressure is the force exerted by the blood against the walls of the blood vessels as it flows through them. Normal BP of healthy individual is 120/80 mm Hg.

ETHICS IN NURSING

Ethics are the rules or principles that govern right conduct. They deal with what is good and bad, and with moral duty and obligation.

TACHYCARDIA

It is increase of pulse rate more than 80 to 100/min.

BACTERIOSTATIC

Agents which halt the progress of bacterias.

RESPIRATION

It is process of exhale or inhale of gas from lungs.

2. a. Discuss the importance of documentation in nursing.
b. Write the various types of records which are used in wards.

IMPORTANCE OF DOCUMENTATION IN NURSING

Refer paper 2008 Q no 3 (a).

TYPES OF RECORDS WHICH ARE USED IN WARDS

Refer paper 2008 Q no 3 (b).

3. a. Define enema.
b. Write the classification of enema.
c. Explain the procedure of soap and water enema.

ENEMA

Enema: An enema is the cleaning of a portion of the large bowel by insertion of fluid rectally.

CLASSIFICATION OF ENEMA

Refer paper 2006 Q no 3 (a).

PROCEDURE OF SOAP AND WATER ENEMA

Refer paper 2006 Q no 3 (b).

4. a. Define nursing.
b. Elaborate the scope of nursing.

NURSING

Nursing is the unique function of the nurse that is to assist the individual in the performance of those activities contributing to health or its recovery, that he would perform unaided if he had the necessary strength, will or knowledge.

SCOPE OF NURSING

Refer paper 2009 Q no 4(a)

5. Write down the purposes on any three of the following:

a. Operation bed
b. Fowler's position
c. Cold compresses
d. Air mattress

OPERATION BED

Refer important theory Q no 5.

FOWLER'S POSITION

Refer important theory Q no 12.

COLD COMPRESSES

Refer paper 2005 Q no 6(e).

Purposes

- To reduce hyperpyrexia
- To decrease the swelling, pain and congestion
- To reduce pain
- To avoid paining sensation
- To relieve muscle spasm.

AIR MATTRESS

- To prevent bed sore
- To prevent pressure on the body
- Useful for bed-ridden patient
- To protect from friction.

6. Write short notes on any three of the following:

a. Qualities of nurse
b. Holistic nursing
c. Care of rubber articles
d. Admission procedure of patient in hospital
e. Comfort devices used in hospital

QUALITIES OF NURSE

Refer paper 2008 Q no 1(b)

HOLISTIC NURSING

- From age old times, nursing is a holistic profession. Many of the nursing theories have explained about the different aspects of holistic nursing. By promoting high-level wellness and preventing illness whenever possible, the holistic nurse uses an approach that minimizes risk and empowers the client. Holistic nurses understand the importance of providing healthy environment for themselves and to the clients.

- Holistic nurse acts as a caring colleague of the client.
- Holistic nurses are aware of the individual responsibility of the clients to choose health and move towards wellness.
- The holistic nurse must keep the whole person in mind when assessing one part of an individual and consider how that part relates to all other parts.
- Holistic health care considers all the components of health, health promotion, health maintenance, health education and illness prevention and rehabilitation care.
- Holistic practitioners advocate the use of lifestyle modification skills such as meditation, exercise or relaxation that alleviate stress and promote a state less susceptible to disease.
- The concept of holistic approach to health is not a new one. It is as old as medicine itself.

CARE OF RUBBER ARTICLES

Refer paper 2006 Q no 4(a).

ADMISSION PROCEDURE OF PATIENT IN HOSPITAL

Admission of a client means, allowing a client to stay in the hospital for observation, investigations and treatment of the disease he is suffering from.

The admission of a client to a hospital can be either emergency or routine. The emergency admission means that the clients are admitted in acute conditions requiring immediate treatment, e.g. clients with heart attack, accidents, poisonings, labor pains, diarrheas, dyspnea, shock, etc.

In emergency admission, every moment is precious. Therefore, the clients should be admitted to the casualty department or emergency ward and the immediate treatment is initiated to save the life of the client.

Routine admission means that the clients are admitted for investigations and planned treatments and surgeries, e.g. the clients with hypertension, diabetes, chronic renal failure, jaundice, hernia, cirrhosis of liver, nephritis, bronchitis, etc.

COMFORT DEVICES USED IN HOSPITAL

Refer paper 2005 Q no 4(b).

Fundamental of Nursing
December 2013

Time: 3 Hours **Maximum Marks: 75**

Note: *Attempt all questions. Please attempt parts of the same question altogether and not in parts.*

1. (a) Define health care team and which are the personnel included in the health care team. **5+5+5 = 15**

(b) Classification of hospitals according to systems.

(c) Explain the functions of hospitals.

2. (a) List the complications of dirty mouth. **5+5+5 = 15**

(b) Explain the causes of bed sores and its signs and symptoms.

(c) Explain the role of nurses in prevention of bed sores.

3. (a) Explain the methods of oxygen administration. **5+5+5 = 15**

(b) Explain the care of unconscious patient.

(c) List the purpose of hot application.

4. (a) List the common sites for accessing pulse. **5+5+5 = 15**

(b) Explain the factors affecting blood pressure.

(c) Convert the 40 degree centigrade into fahrenheit.

5. Write short notes on any three of the following: **5+5+5 = 15**

(a) Comfort devices

(b) Role of nurse in disaster management

(c) Rigor

(d) Care of rubber articles

(e) Bandaging

SOLVED PAPER DECEMBER 2013

1. (a) Define health care team and which are the personnel included in the health care team.

(b) Classification of hospitals according to systems.

(c) Explain the functions of hospitals.

HEALTH CARE TEAM

The health care team consists of a group of people who coordinate their particular skills in order to assist a client or his family. The personal included in the health team are as follows:

- **The physician:** A phsician is responsible for the medical diagnosis and for determining the therapy required by a person who is ill or injured.
- **Nursing team:** Composed of personnel who provide nursing services to a client or his family. The team leader is responsible for the delegation of duties to the members of her team and the care given to the clients.
- **The dietitians or nutritionist:** May be a members of the health team. Dietitians design special diets and they supervise the preparations of the meals according to the needs of the client and according to the doctors prescription.
- **Physiotherapist:** Provides assistance to a client who has problems related to his musculoskeletal system.
- **Occupational therapist:** Assists clients with some impairment of functions to gain skills as they relate to activities of daily living.
- **The pharmacist:** Who prepares and dispenses medicines in the hospital and community settings.
- Social worker assists the clients with such problems like finances.
- Non professional workers are also sometimes included in the health team since they meet the needs of the client.

CLASSIFICATION OF HOSPITALS

Refer important theory question no 19 page no 8–9

FUNCTIONS OF HOSPITAL

Refer paper 2005 question no 6 (d)

2. (a) List the complications of dirty mouth.
(b) Explain the causes of bed sores and its signs and symptoms.
(c) Explain the role of nurses in prevention of bed sores.

COMPLICATIONS OF DIRTY MOUTH

- **Halitosis:** It is the offensive odor of breath.
- **Dental caries:** It is a destructive process causing decalcification of the enamel and dentin with resulting cavitation of the tooth.
- **Dental plaque:** It is a soft thin film of food debris, mucin and dead epithelial cells that is deposited on the teeth.

- **Pyorrhea:** It is the pus formation in the sockets of the teeth.
- **Sordes:** Brown crusts which are formed on the teeth and lips.
- **Cheilosis:** It is the cracking or ulceration of the lips and angles of the mouth.
- **Bleeding gums:** It occur in vitamin C deficiency, use hard brush.
- **Glossitis:** It is an inflammation of the tongue.
- **Root abscess:** It is pus formation in the root of the teeth.
- **Stomatitis:** It is the inflammation of the mucous membrane of the mouth.

CAUSES AND SIGNS AND SYMPTOMS OF BED SORES

Refer paper 2007 question no 2 (a)

ROLE OF NURSES IN PREVENTION OF BED SORES

Refer paper 2007 question no 2 (a)

3. (a) Explain the methods of oxygen administration.
(b) Explain the care of unconscious patient.
(c) List the purpose of hot application.

METHODS OF OXYGEN ADMINISTRATION

- **Oxygen by nasal catheter:** It is most common method of administering O_2 to the patients in hospital wards. The nasal catheter is inserted into the nostril reaching up to the uvula and is held in place by adhesive tapes. Flow of 1 to 4 liters of oxygen will be sufficient to maintain the concentration of 22 to 30% oxygen.
- **Oxygen by mask:** A variety of face masks that cover the patient's nose and mouth are available for oxygen administration. If the mask does not fit snugly over the face, O_2 lost from the masks. Masks are advantageous for those patients who are unable to breathe through the nose.
- **Oxygen tent:** An oxygen tent consists of a canopy over the patient fully or partially and it is connected to a supply of oxygen. The canopies are transparent and enable the nurses to observe the patient. The lower part of the canopy is tucked under the bed to prevent the escape of oxygen.

CARE OF UNCONSCIOUS PATIENT

Nursing diagnosis: Ineffective airway clearance:

- Assess respiratory rate pattern, lung sounds, lung expansion, signs of tissue, hypoxia, cyanosis, pallor, presence of airway secretion.

- Elevate head of bed to 30° or place client in lateral or semiprone position.
- Insert oral airway.
- Suction airway intermittently.
- Connect the client to mechanical ventilator as needed.
- Increase amount of fluids administered at least 2.5 liter per day.
- Auscultate chest at least every 8 hours.
- Monitor arterial blood gas (ABG) measurements.

Nursing diagnosis: Ineffective cerebral tissue perfusion:

- Assess signs of increased intracranial pressure (ICP), cerebral edema.
- Maintain head of the bed elevated to 30°.
- Administer low flow oxygen.
- Suction airway when needed.
- Maintain patent airway.

Nursing diagnosis: Risk for injury related to unconscious state:

- Assess the risk factors for injury, e.g. lack of side rails, etc.
- Keep side rails up and bed in lowest position
- Use padded side rails
- Keep clients nail short
- Administer prescribed seizure drugs.
- Always turn the client toward the nurse.
- Protect from external sources of heat such as hot water bags.
- Avoid over sedation.

Nursing diagnosis: Risk for impaired tissue integrity (cornea) related to absence of corneal blink, reflex and dryness of eyes:

- Assess signs of impaired corneal integrity.
- Protect eyes with an eye shield.
- Inspect the condition of eyes with a flash light at regular intervals.
- Remove contact lenses if any.
- Irrigate eyes with sterile saline.

Nursing diagnosis: Imbalance nutrition:

- Assess nutritional status
- Administer fluids IV
- Administer fluid diet in the form of juice, shake, soup, water via Ryle's tube.
- Start total parenteral nutrition (TPN), if the client cannot tolerate Ryle's tube.
- Record parameters such as weight, height and lab test at regular intervals.

PURPOSE OF HOT APPLICATION

- To relieve pain
- To relieve congestion
- To provide warmth
- To promote suppuration
- To promote healing
- To decrease muscle tone
- To soften the exudates.

4. (a) List the common sites for accessing pulse.
(b) Explain the factors affecting blood pressure.
(c) Convert the 40 degree centigrade into fahrenheit.

COMMON SITES FOR ACCESSING PULSE

Refer paper 2006 question no 2 (b)

FACTORS AFFECTING BLOOD PRESSURE (BP)

- **Age:** BP is lower in children than in adults.
- **Sex:** Before puberty their is no difference in boys and girls BP.
- **Race:** Certain races, e.g. Negroes will have higher BP reading than other races.
- **Climate:** Pressure norms are lower in tropical climates than temperate and highest in polar climates.
- **Times of the day:** In all persons, BP is lowest in the early morning and then rises to a peak in the evening.
- **Exercise:** Muscular exertion will raise the BP.
- **Pain:** Severe pain may cause temporary and marked increase in the BP.
- **Emotion:** Fear, worry, excitement and other emotional factors will raise the BP.
- **Posture:** BP is lower when lying down then sitting or standing.
- **Drugs:** The drugs such as amyl nitrite and nitroglycerin cause decrease in the BP. Certain drugs increase the BP.
- **Disease conditions:** Diseases affecting the circulatory system and kidneys may increase BP.
- **Hemorrhage:** It causes low BP by decreasing the volume of blood.
- **Increased intracranial pressure:** Pressure in the cranium usually produce a rise in the BP, e.g. head injury and intracranial tumors.

CONVERT 40 °C TO °F

$$F = \left(C \times \frac{9}{5}\right) + 32$$

$$F = \left(\overset{8}{\cancel{40}} \times \frac{9}{\cancel{5}}\right) + 32$$

$$F = 72 + 32 = 104$$

$$= 104\ °F$$

5. Write short notes on any three of the following:

(a) Comfort devices
(b) Role of nurse in disaster management
(c) Rigor
(d) Care of rubber articles
(e) Bandaging

COMFORT DEVICES

Refer paper 2005 question no 4 (b)

ROLE OF NURSE IN DISASTER MANAGEMENT

Each locality has its own standard operating procedure for disaster operations. But in general following procedure can help:

- A command post is established in a safe area.
- Communication is to be established with hospitals, medical facilities, dispatchers and other emergency units.
- Hazards control must begin as soon as possible. These must be close coordination between rescue personnel, fire fighters and low enforcement officers.
- A triage point should be set up in safe area in such a way so that al patients are funnelled through triage before they are taken to ambulance for transport.
- When possible patients are removed according to the severity of their injuries but this is not always practical.
- All ambulance drivers should stay with their vehicles. First aider should report to triage officer along with equipment.
- The command post should determine the hospital to which a particular ambulance should go.
- A special care area should be set up to receive relatives and friends of the disaster victims, person incharge of this area must make certain that only reliable information is passed on to friends and relatives.
- Emergency care should be available at the information center.

- Dead bodies may not be removed from the scene until all the injured patients have been transported.

RIGOR

Refer paper 2005 question no 1 (j)

CARE OF RUBBER ARTICLES

Refer paper 2006 question no 4 (a)

BANDAGING

It is the protective covering of a wound.

Purposes

- To prevent infection.
- To prevent further complications.
- To absorb any blood or discharge.
- To promote healing.

Points to Remember while Bandaging

- The bandage should be done in neat, clean manner and it should be dry.
- Width of bandage and length of bandage.
- The bandage should not be too tight and not too loose.
- Pressure bandage should be able to stop bleeding.
- The bandage should cover completely the dressing material.
- Put some cotton wool on the part to be bandaged so that the bandage does not slip or cause cutting into the skin underneath.
- Hold the head of bandage in right hand.
- Don't tie or put knot over the wound.
- Instruct the patient how to prevent bandage from soiling.
- Avoid covering the nail to check the circulation of the area.
- Secure the bandage properly with adhesive material.
- Never use wrinkled bandage.
- Listen to all the complaints of patient while bandaging.

Types

According to the size and shape of bandages, they are:
- Roller bandages
- Binders

- Many tailed bandages
- T-bandage
- Tubular gauze
- Simple spiral
- Figure of eight
- Reverse spiral
- Spiral bandage
- Triangular bandage.

Fundamental of Nursing
January 2013

Time: 3 Hours **Maximum Marks: 75**

Note: *Attempt all questions. Attempt all parts of questions in continuity*

1. Define the following:
(a) Tachycardia
(b) Anorexia
(c) Asepsis
(d) Nursing
(e) Insomnia
(f) Sterilizatiion
(g) Bedsore
(h) Disinfectant
(i) Blood Pressure
(j) Fever **10×1=10**

2. Write down the purposes of any three of the following:
(a) Mouth care
(b) Hot water bottle
(c) Bed making
(d) Soap and water enema **3×5=15**

3. Discuss the role of nurse in three of the following:
(a) Care of patient with high fever
(b) Collection of specimen
(c) Care of dying patient
(d) Care of patient with communication disease. **3×5=15**

4. Explain any three of the following:
(a) Five rights for administering the drug
(b) Care of pressure points
(c) Steps to reduce nosocomial infection in the hospital
(d) Contraindications of oral medication. **3×5=15**

5. Write short notes on any four of the following:
(a) Holistic nursing
(b) Shock
(c) Functions of the hospital
(d) Hot and cold applications
(e) Qualities of nurse **4×5=20**

SOLVED QUESTION PAPER 2013

1. Define the following:

(a) Tachycardia
(b) Anorexia
(c) Asepsis
(d) Nursing
(e) Insomnia
(f) Sterilizatiion
(g) Bedsore
(h) Disinfectant
(i) Blood pressure
(j) Fever

TACHYCARDIA

A pulse rate over 100/min is called tachycardia.

ANOREXIA

It means loss of appetite.

ASEPSIS

Freedom from infections or prevention of contact with microorganisms.

NURSING

Nursing is a dynamic, therapeutic and educative process in meeting the health needs of the individual family and society.

INSOMNIA

It is defined as the inability to sleep or it is a lessening of the duration of depth of sleep.

STERILIZATION

It is the destruction of all the microorganisms both pathogenic and non-pathogenic including their spares.

BEDSORE

It is known as decubitus ulcers. It occur due to pressure from lying on matte or sitting on a chair for a prolonged period of time resulting in the slowing of circulations and finally death of tissues.

DISINFECTANT

An agent which kills pathogenic organisms. It is applied particularly to agents used on an animate objects.

BLOOD PRESSURE

BP is the force created by the blood against the walls of the blood vessels at it flow through them. Normal BP of healthy individual is 120/80 mm Hg.

FEVER

Fever or pyrexia is defined as a rise in the body temperature about 99°F.

2. Write down the purposes of any three of the following:

(a) Mouth care (b) Hot water bottle

(c) Bed making (d) Soap and water enema

MOUTH CARE

Refer Paper September 2005 Q. No. 2(b)

HOT WATER BOTTLE

- To stimulate circulation
- To promote suppuration
- To promote healing
- To relieve pain
- To reduce inflammation and congestion
- To supply warmth and comfort
- To relieve muscle spasm
- To relieve retention of urine.

BED MAKING

- Provide the client with a safe and comfortable bed to take rest and sleep.
- To give to the unit or ward a neat apearance
- To adopt to the needs of the client and to be ready for any emergency.
- To economize time, material and effort.
- To prevent bedsore.
- To promote cleanliness
- To establish an effective nurse client relationship.
- To provide active and passive exercise to the clients.
- To help the relations to learn to care for the sick at home.

SOAP AND WATER ENEMA

Refer 2005, Q. No. 2(a)

3. Discuss the role of nurse in three of the following:
(a) Care of patient with high fever
(b) Collection of specimen
(c) Care of dying patient
(d) Care of patient with communication disease.

CARE OF POTENTIAL WITH HIGH FEVER

Refer Paper 2005 Q. No. 5

COLLECTION OF SPECIMEN

Refer Important Theory Q. No. 8

CARE OF DYING PATIENT

Refer Paper 2009 Q. 3(b)

CARE OF PATIENT WITH COMMUNICABLE DISEASE

- Barrier nursing or isolation technique is used for the care of patient with communicable disease. There are number of isolation techniques and precautions used to prevent spread of infection.
- Respiratory isolation
- Enteric isolation
- Wound and skin isolation
- Blood isolation.

General Precautions

- Maintain a high degree of cleanliness.
- **Health Teching:** Client and his relatives are to be taught about the spread of infection and its prevention.
- Minimize the numbers of visitors
- Emphasize on hand washing wash hands after elimination before eating and after handling the client or his articles.
- Keep toilet articles separate for each person.
- As far as possible, the clients should be separate room.
- If separate rooms are not available there should be at least a sufficient space in between the beds.
- Wash hand thoroughly.
- Nurse who provide care to the patient also wear proper gown, gloves and mask.

- The gown is worn by the infected person when he is transported outside his room. The gown prevents the clients contaminated clothing from touching clean areas.
- Put on the 'clean' gloves.

4. Explain any three of the following:

(a) Five rights for administering the drug

(b) Care of pressure points

(c) Steps to reduce nosocomial infection in the hospital

(d) Contraindications of oral medication.

FIVE RIGHTS FOR ADMINISTERING THE DRUG

Right Client

- Read the physicians orders to make sure for whom the medicine is ordered.
- Read the client's name on the client's chart and on the medicine chart.
- Call the client by name and ask him to repeat his name.

Right Drug

- Read the physician's orders to study the correct name of the drug.
- To make sure the drug is copied correctly on the medicine card, on the nurse's record, etc.
- Be careful of drugs whose name sound alike.
- Select the right drugs from cupboard. Read the label of the medicine container and name of the medicine in the medicine card thrice.
- Look for the color, odor, and consistency of the drug.
- Administer medicine only from a clearly labeled containers.
- Be familiar with the trade names of doubt consult the phjysician or medicine book.
- Avoid accepting the verbal orders.
- Always identifying the client before giving medication.
- Make sure that the drug has not been discontinued by the physician.

Right Dose

- Read the physician's orders to know the correct dose.
- Consider the age and weight of the client. This may help to find an error in the physician's orders.
- Know the minimum of maximum dose of the medicine administered.

- Measure accurately.
- Have the medicine card or written order in hand before you prepare the drug.
- Consider how many tablets or capsules are required for the dose.
- Know the abbreviations and symbols used.
- Help the client to take all medicine that is ordered.
- The medicine should be carried to the client without spilling it out of the container.

Right Time

- Read the physician's orders.
- Know the hospital routines for the intervals.
- Give at started intervals for blood levels.
- Know the abbreviations for the time, e.g. BD, TDS, etc.
- Give the medicine at proper time.
- Give the medicine as ordered in relation to the food intake, e.g., before food or after food.
- Give medicine according to the action excepted, e.g. sleeping pills are given at bed time.

Right Method

- Read the physician's order.
- Dilute the medicine, if indicated.
- Know the method of giving drugs, e.g. orally, parenterally, rectally, etc.
- Know the abbreviations such as IM, IV, PO, etc.
- Identify the client correctly.
- Stay with the client until he/she has taken the medication.
- Never leave the client medicine with the client
- An error in the medication should be reported immediately.

CARE OF PRESSURE POINTS

Refer 2010, Q. No. 1(b).

PREVENTION OF NOSOCOMIAL INFECTION IN THE HOSPITAL

Refer Important Theory Q. No. 2.

CONTRAINDICATION OF ORAL MEDICATION

Refer paper 2007 Q. No. 2f.

5. Write short notes on any four of the following:

(a) Holistic nursing (b) Shock

(c) Functions of the hospital (d) Hot and cold applications

(e) Qualities of nurse

HOLISTIC NURSING

From age old times, nursing is a holistic profession. Many of the nursing theories have explained about the different aspects of holistic nursing. By promoting high level wellness and preventing illness. Whenever possible, the holistic nurse uses an approach that minimizes risk and empower the client.

Holistic nurse understand the importance of providing healthy environment for themselves and to the client. The holistic nurse must keep the wholesale person in mind. When assessing one part of an individual and consider how that part relates to all other parts. The nurse must also consider how the individual interacts with and relates to the external environment and to others.

Holistic practitioners advocate the use of lifestyle modification skills such as meditation, exercise or relaxation that alleviate stress and promote a state less susceptible to diseases.

The concept of holistic approach to health is not a new one. It is as old as medicine itself.

SHOCK

Refer Paper 2008, Q. No. 5b.

FUNCTIONS OF THE HOSPITAL

Refer Paper 2005, Q.No. 6(d).

HOT AND COLD APPLICATIONS

Hot Applications

It is the application of a hot agent, warmer than skin either in a moist or dry form on the surface of the body to relieve pain and congestion, to provide warmth, to promote suppuration to promote healing, to decrease muscle tone and to soften the excudates.

Classification of Hot Applications

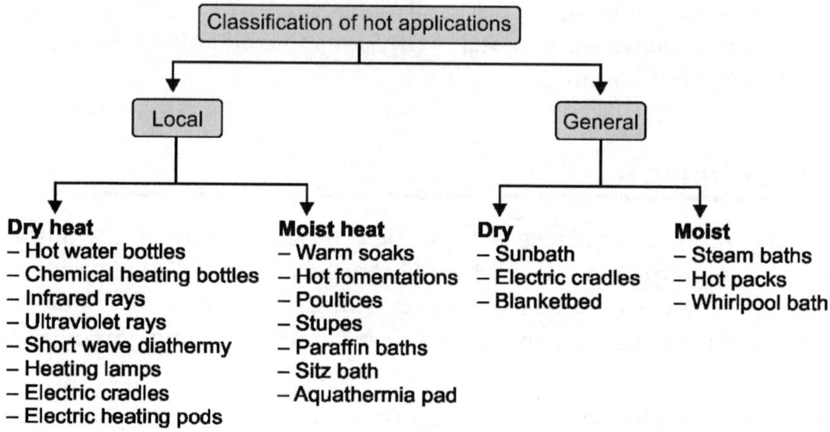

Cold Applications

Cold applications is the application of a cold agent cooler than skin either in a moist or dry from on the surface of the skin, to reduce pain and body temperature, to anesthetize an area, to check haemorrhage, to prevent gangrene to prevent edema, and reduce inflammation.

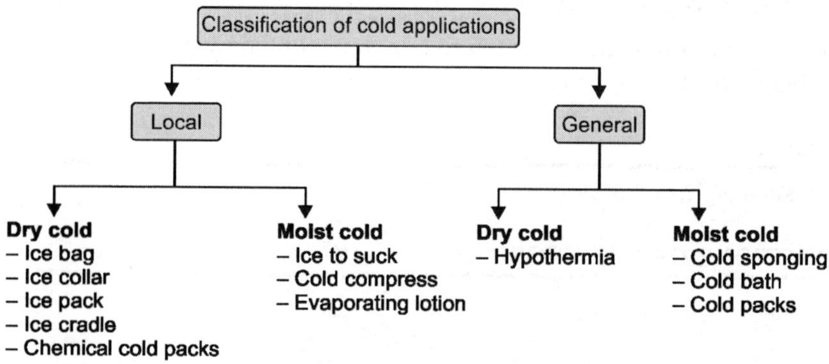

QUALITIES OF NURSE

Refer Paper 2008, Q. No. 1(b).

Fundamental of Nursing
January 2012

Time: 3 Hours | **Maximum Marks: 75**

Note: *Attempt all the questions. Attempt all parts of question at same place.*

1. Define the following terms:

(a) Asepsis
(b) Hyperpyrexia
(c) Ethics
(d) Sitz bath
(e) Hypertension
(f) Nursing
(g) Isolation
(h) Intermittent fever
(i) Sterilization
(j) Personal hygiene **1×10=10**

2. Elaborate the role of nurse in following (any two):

(a) Drug administration
(b) While giving enema
(c) Discharge of a patient **2×5=10**

3. (a) Define decubitus ulcer.

(b) What are common sites of decubitus ulcer and the causes of decubitus ulcer?

(c) Discuss the prevention and management of decubitus ulcer.

2+8+10=20

4. Write down purposes of the following:

(a) Back care
(b) Ice-cap
(c) Oral hygiene
(d) Steam inhalation
(e) Admission bed **5×3=15**

5. Write a short note on any five:

(a) Range of motion (ROM)
(b) First aid of burn case
(c) Determinants of health
(d) Nursing care in high fever
(e) Principles of records
(f) Nursing process **5×4=20**

SOLVED QUESTION PAPER 2012

1. Define the following terms.

(a) Asepsis
(b) Hyperpyrexia
(c) Ethics
(d) Sitz bath
(e) Hypertension
(f) Nursing
(g) Isolation
(h) Intermittent fever
(i) Sterilization
(j) Personal hygiene

ASEPSIS

Freedom from infection or prevention of contact with microorganisms.

HYPERPYREXIA

The temperature goes above 105°F.

ETHICS

Ethics are the rules or principles that govern right conduct. They deal with what is good and bad, and with moral duty and obligation. Ethics are designed to protect the rights of human beings.

SITZ BATH

It is method of applying heat using tepid or hot water to the pelvic or rectal area by sitting in a tub, or special chair or basin filled with sufficient water to reach the umbilicus.

HYPERTENSION

It is blood pressure that is above normal for a sustained period.

NURSING

Nursing is a dynamic, therapeutic and educative process in meeting the health needs of the individual, family and society.

ISOLATION

It is the separation of infected person from the non-infected person for the period of communicability under conditions which will prevent the transmission of infection to others.

INTERMITTENT FEVER

The temperature rises from normal or subnormal to high fever and back at regular intervals. The interval may vary from few hours to 3 days. Usually, the temperature is higher in the evening than in the morning.

STERILIZATION

It is the destruction of all the microorganisms both pathogenic and non-pathogenic including their spores.

PERSONAL HYGIENE

Personal hygiene refers to maintenance of cleanliness of our body.

2. Elaborate the role of nurse in following (any two):

(a) Drug administration
(b) While giving enema
(c) Discharge of a patient.

DRUG ADMINISTRATION

Ans. *Refer Paper 2008 Q. No. 4a.*

ROLE OF NURSE WHILE GIVING ENEMA

Preliminary Assessment

- Check the diagnosis.
- Check the date and type of surgery.
- Check the consciousness and the ability to follow direction.
- Check the abilities and limitations concerning movement.
- Check the nature of enema ordered and special precautions, if any to be followed.
- Check the general condition of the client and the ability to retain the fluid.
- Check the medical order for the collection of stool specimens if any, for laboratory tests.
- Check for any lesions on the rectal and perineal area.
- Any extra help needed, e.g. to place the bedpan in position.
- Articles available in the client's unit.

Preparation of the Client and the Unit

- Explain the procedure to the client to win his confidence and cooperation. explain the discomfort caused by the enema fluid and need for retaining the solution for sometime.
- Provide privacy with curtains.
- Cover the client with a sheet or bath blanket and fanfold the top linen to the foot end of the bed.
- Remove the backrest and pillows.
- Place the Mackintosh and towel under the client's buttocks to protect the bed and the linen.
- Place the client in a left lateral position with the buttock close to the edge of the bed.
- Keep all articles arranged on the bedside locker.
- Keep the bedpan under the bed over a paper or stool.
- Adjust the IV pole or overbed table to hold the enema can at the required height.
- Remove bottom garments or raise it above the waist level.
- Drape the client immediately before giving the enema. Fold back a small portion of the sheet or the bath blanket, covering the client to expose only the anus.

After Care of the Client and Articles

- Encourage the client to retain the fluid for 10 to 15 minutes. Encourage slow breathing with open mouth for relaxation.
- Turn the client on the back and assist him onto toilet, commode or bedpan.
- Give a call signal to the client and leave him alone for sometime if safe.
- Observe enema results, nothing the color, consistency and the amount, obtain specimens if desired.
- Bring the toilet tray and assist him for perineal care.
- Remove the bedpan, dry the client, put on the garments, change the bed linen if needed, straighten the sheets and adjust the position of the client in the bed to make him comfortable.
- Explain the client that he may need to evacuate the bowel several times in the next few hours.
- Take the bedpan to the sanitary annex, inspect the contents empty the bedpan clean it and keep it on the bedpan rack for the next use.
- Take all articles to the utility room.
- Wash hands.

- Records the types of enema, the result, with the date and time on the nurse's record.
- Evaluate the client's condition and comfort.
- Send the specimen, if any to the laboratory.

DISCHARGE OF A PATIENT

Preparation of the Client for Discharge

Rehabilitation of the Client

No client should be discharged until he is rehabilitated. The rehabilitation begins when a client first comes in contact with the health care team. A nurse is concerned with facilitating optimal independence for a client whether the client is experiencing a short-term illness or long-term illness.

Planning for the Client's Discharge

- A suitable day fixed for the termination of care in the hospital.
- **Explain** the relatives, so that they could prepare to take the client home.
- Some of the nursing procedure's, which the client may have to continue at home, should be taught to him or his family members who will be caring for him at home.
- Give instruction and explanation or instruction to client about treatment, diet, exercise or medications.
- Demonstrated to the client and made familiar with the type of diet he has to continue at home.
- Watch for the reaction of the client about discharge.
- The nurse give psychological support to the clients.
- The nurse may explain to the relatives about the physical and mental changes due to illness.

Discharge Procedure

- No client should be discharged without the doctor's written order.
- Instructions regarding further care, medication treatment, follow-up, etc. should be clearly written and interpreted to the client and to his family members.
- All the belongings such as clothing, money and other valuables returned to him.
- The articles in the clients unit should be checked and see that they are complete including the bed lines.

- Before the client leave the hospital, the nurse should confirm whether he has paid all the hospital bills.
- See that the client is ready to go home, recently bathed, hair combed and dressed in clean clothes.
- If the client is not able to walk or not allowed to walk to the conveyance the nurse should see that he is safety transferred either on a wheelchair or on a stretcher.
- The diatary department should be informed of the client's discharge.
- The nurses should see that the charts are completed and sent to the officer or to the record section to be filled.

Care of the Unit after Discharge of Client

- The room should be cleaned and aired, windows and doors are opened.
- The doors, windows, furniture are washed and cleaned.
- All articles used by client should be taken to the utility room.
- All unwanted things are discarded.
- If the room was used for a communicable disease, it should be fumigated with articles used by the client.

3. (a) Define decubitus ulcer.

(b) What are common sites of decubitus ulcer and the causes of decubitus ulcer?

(c) Discuss the prevention and management of decubitus ulcer.

Ans. *Refer Paper 2007 Q. No. 2a.*

4. Write down purposes of the following:

(a) Back care (b) Ice-cap

(c) Oral hygiene (d) Steam inhalation

(e) Admission bed

BACK CARE

- To clean the body off dirt and Bacteria
- To increase elimination through the skin
- To prevent bedsores
- To stimulate circulation
- To induce sleep
- To provide comfort to the patient
- To relieve fatigue
- To give the patient a sense of well-being
- To regulate body temperature
- To observe objective symptoms

- To give the nurse an opportunity for healthy teaching
- To establish an effective nurse patient relationship.

PURPOSES OF ICE-CAP

- To reduce hyperpyrexia
- To decrease the swelling and pain, congestion
- To reduce pain
- To avoid paining sensation
- To relieve muscle spasm.

ORAL HYGIENE

- To feel fresh
- To prevent infection
- To increase blood circulation
- To stimulate appetite
- To remove the dirt and growth of bacteria
- To give the sense of well-being
- To prevent the complication arising in the neglected mouth
- To clean mouth of helpless patients very sick and unconscious patients.

STEAM INHALATION

- To relieve the inflammation of congestion of the mucous membrane of respiratory tract
- To soften the thick and tenacious secretion
- To provide moisture heat and prevent dryness of the mucous membrane of respiratory tract
- To relieve spasm of larynx and bronchi
- To apply antiseptic action by use of menthol, TR Benz Co.

ADMISSION BED

- Admission bed is prepared for a new admission patient
- To clean the patient
- To observe the patient head to toe
- To provide comfort to the patient
- To help the physician to do the physical examination.

5. Write a short note on any five:

(a) Range of motion (ROM)

(b) First aid of burn case

(c) Determinants of health
(d) Nursing care in high fever
(e) Principles of records
(f) Nursing process

RANGE OF MOTION

The range of motion is directly concerned with the active and passive exercises. They plays an important role in perfect completion of different nursing procedures in caring the patient. The range of motion is associated with principles of physics making a nurse more comfortable and less tiring while doing nursing procedures in the wards. By adopting accurate scientific principles a nurse works more effectively saving her time and efforts.

FIRST AID OF BURN CASE

Refer Paper 2007 Q. No. 2(c).

DETERMINANTS OF HEALTH

Health is multifactor. The health of individual and community is result of man-interactions. The genetic factors and environmental factors affect the health. Some important determinants of health are given below:

- Heredity
- Environment
- Lifestyle
- Socioeconomic status
- Health and family welfare services
- Other factor.

Heredity

The physical and mental traits of every human being are determined by nature of genes at the times of conception. The genetic make-up cannot be altered after conception and number of diseases are genetic origin, e.g. chromosomal abnormalities, mental retardation, sometimes diabetes and metabolic disease.

Environment

Environment is classified as internal and external; and internal environment pertains to every tissue, organ system and harmonious functioning wise in the system. External environment consists of factors to which man is exposed to after coming in contact with external environment, i.e. after birth it affects physical, mental, social well-being of person. The environmental, factors are housing, water supply, psychosocial stress, etc.

Lifestyle

The term lifestyle denotes to the concept, the way people live. It reflects to the social values attitude and activities. It includes cultural or behavioral pattern and life long personal habit. Health needs promotion of healthy lifestyle in developing countries. The current health problem, e.g. coronary artery disease, obesity, lung cancer, drug addiction are closely related to lifestyle changes in developing countries, the richness and illness and health are connected in the lack of sanitation and poor nutrition personal hygiene, human habits, customs and cultural patterns.

Socioeconomic Conditions

It have great inpact on human health. Health status is determined by total income, education nutrition, employment, housing, etc. The optimum health demand lifestyle should be the aim of every individual. It plays an important role in reducing morbidity increases life expectancy and improving lifestyle. Education and occupation also play important role in this.

Health Services

Health of family depends upon health care services provided. They work for prevention of disease and promotion of health. Better health services promotes health status, e.g. immunization influence the prevalence of disease.

Other Factor

Other factors contributing of health of population are from outside the health care system, i.e. food and agriculture, industries, social welfare, rural development, employment opportunities, increased wages, prepaid medical programs and family support system, etc.

NURSING CARE IN HIGH FEVER

Refer Paper 2005 Q. No. 5(c).

PRINCIPLES OF RECORDS

Principles of records are following:

- **Date and time:** Document the date and time of each recording. Record the time in the conventional manner, e.g. 9 am to 3 pm, etc. This is important not only due to legal reasons but also for the clients safety.
- **Correct spelling:** It is essential for accuracy in recording. In case of doubt, check the dictionary and use the correct spelling.
- **Appropriateness:** Record only information that pertains to the client's health problems and care.
- **Legal prudence:** Accurate complete documentation give legal protection to the nurse, other health care professional of the institution and the client.
- **Accuracy:** Clients's name and identification data must be written on each page of the clinical record. Entries must be accurate.
- **Completeness:** Document all information necessary to explain the events in a shift. Anyone reading the document should have a clear picture of what took place or is being described. Complete pertinent assessment data such as vital signs, wound drainage, client's complaints, who was notified and what interventions were carried out, give a complete picture, so that nurses on subsequent shift can make objective evaluations and revise the plan as headed. Include the following information in the chart:
  - Any now or changed information
  - Signs and symptoms
  - Client behavior
  - Nursing intervention
  - Medication given
  - Physician's orders carried out
  - Client teaching
  - Client response.
- **Conciseness and brevity:** Good charting is concise and brief. Use partial sentences and phases, drop the client's name and terms referring to the client use only accepted abbreviations, which are approved by the particular health care facility.
- **Legibility:** Writing must be clear and easily readable by others. Legibility is all the more important while recording numbers and medical terms.
- **Organization:** Recording of information on the Client's record must follow a chronological order. Charting statements must be logically organized according to time and content.
- **Sequence and timeliness:** Documentation in a timely manner can help avoid errors. Record all medications at the time they are given procedures, treatment and assessments should be recorded as soon as possible

after their completion timeliness helps to avoid forgetting important information.

- **Correction:** Two types of corrections made to a record are, correcting a written entry and adding an entry later. When an error occurs do not erase it.
- **Omissions:** Blank space are not be left on the chart. Avoid writing outside the lines of the charting format. A horizontal line is drawn through any empty space to the right margin to prevent later entries being made in front of a signature.
- **Signature:** A written signature must follow every entry into a client's record. The correct way to sign a notation is using the first initial and full last name followed by the abbreviation of the health care workers position title, e.g. RNRM.
- **Confidentiality:** Records of client should not be discussed with any 3rd party. It should be kept confidential, not shown and handover any outside person other than care provider.

NURSING PROCESS

Refer Paper 2010 Q. No. – 3 (a, b).

Fundamental of Nursing
November 2010

Time: 3 Hours | *Maximum Marks: 75*

Note: *Attempt all questions.*

1. **Define the following terms:** 10×1 = 10
   (a) Disinfection
   (b) Pressure points
   (c) Comprehensive nursing care
   (d) Inhalation
   (e) Blood pressure
   (f) Fomentation
   (g) Prone position
   (h) Antiseptic solution
   (i) Posture
   (j) Vitamins
2. **Write down the purpose of:** 3×5 = 15
   (a) Checking vital signs
   (b) Urine analysis
3. **Explain the following:**
   (a) What is a nursing process? 3
   (b) What are the steps of nursing care plan? 5
   (c) Make a nursing care plan of a patient with respiratory infection. 12
4. **Write short notes on any three:** 3×5 = 15
   (a) First aid in insect bite.
   (b) Role of nurse in caring of patient with poisoning.
   (c) splinting a leg with fracture.
   (d) Emergency care in rod accident.
   (e) Analgesics.
5. **(a) 1. List two purposes of exercising.** 2
   2. List two steps to reduce nosocomial infection in the hospital. 2
   3. List two rich sources of carbohydrates. 2

4. Write the full form of: ½ ×4 = 2

(i) NPO (ii) Cap

(iii) IV (iv) SC

(b) Write whether the statements are 'True' or 'False': 7×1 = 7

1. The normal range of pulse is 100–120/min.
2. Savlon is an antifungal agent.
3. Chest physiotherapy helps to dislodge the secretions in the chest.
4. The eye is cleaned from the outer canthus to the inner canthus.
5. Any systemic infection can raise the body temperature.
6. Sodium hypochlorite solution is effective if it is prepared daily.
7. Cyanosis is a good sign in the assessment of clients progress.

SOLVED QUESTION PAPER 2010

1. Define the following terms:

(a) Disinfection
(b) Pressure points
(c) Comprehensive nursing care
(d) Inhalation
(e) Blood pressure
(f) Fomentation
(g) Prone position
(h) Antiseptic solution
(i) Posture
(j) Vitamins

DISINFECTION

It is the process in which all pathogenic organisms are destroyed is known as disinfection.

PRESSURE POINTS

It is also known as decubitus ulcers. It is occur due to pressure from lying on matters or sitting on a chair for a prolonged period of time resulting in the slowing of circulation and finally death of tissues.

COMPREHENSIVE NURSING CARE

It is a systemic process of problem diagnosis, problem analysis, development of plan of care and continuous assessment of evolving plan of care.

INHALATION

Inhalation is the deep breathing of vapor, air or gas into the lungs for a local effect on the air passages or for a systemic effect, e.g. relief of bronchial spasms.

BLOOD PRESSURE

It is the force exerted by the blood against the walls of the blood vessels as it flows through them.

FOMENTATION

Fomentation are moist applications of heat over an area by means of double thickness of flannel or other soft material wring out from hot water, protected by a waterproof covering, wood and bandage.

PRONE POSITION

The client lie flat on the abdomen with head turned to one side. The head rests on a pillow. One or both arms rest in a comfortable way either beyond the head or at the sides of the head.

ANTISEPTIC SOLUTION

A substance that inhibits the growth of bacteria.

POSTURE

It is the way in which the body parts are aligned with one another. It is defined as the position in which the various parts of the body are held when sitting, standing, walking and lying down.

VITAMINS

Vitamins are complex chemical substance. They are required by the body in very small amounts.

2. Write down the purposes of:

(a) Checking vital signs
(b) Using gloves
(c) Urine analysis

CHECKING VITAL SIGNS

- To determine change in clients status.
- To recognize variation from normal and its significance.
- To help physician to prescribe right treatment.

PURPOSES OF USING GLOVES

- To reducing the risks of transmission of microorgnisms.
- To provide a protective barrier.
- To prevent gross contamination of the hands when touching blood, body fluids, secretion, etc.
- To reduce the risk of exposure to blood borne pathogens.

PURPOSES OF URINE ANALYSIS

- To tests the ability to concentrate solutes in the urine.
- To measure the pH level. Normally it is 4.6 to 7.5.
- To measure the specific gravity range from 1.005 to 1.030.
- To assess the color and odor of urine.
- To assess the appearance of urine.
- To find out the any kidney problem like, renal failure, kidney stone, and urine culture, etc.

3. Explain the following:

(a) What is a nursing process?
(b) What are the steps of nursing care plan?
(c) Make a nursing care plan of a patient with respiratory infection.

DEFINE NURSING PROCESS

It is a set of actions used to determine plan, implement and evaluates nursing care.

STEPS OF NURSING CARE PLAN

- Nursing diagnosis
- Planning nursing care
- Scientific rational.
- Expected outcome
- Implementation nursing care

NURSING DIAGNOSIS

- **According to NANDA:** A clinical judgment about individual family, or community responses to actual and potential health processes. Nursing diagnosis provides the basis for selection of nursing intervention to achieve outcomes for which the nurse is accountable.
- **Expected outcome:** Expected outcome describe the behavior, the patient is expected to achieve.
- **Planning nursing care:** Planning is defined as the selecting and carrying out of series of action assigned to achieve stated goals.

- **Implementation:** A nursing intervention is a single nursing action treatment procedure or activity- designed to achieve an outcome to a diagnosis–nursing or medical for which the nurse is accountable.

S. No.	Nursing Diagnosis	Objectives	Planning	Implementation	Evaluation
1.	Impaired gas exchange and airway clearance due to respiratory infection.	To improvement in gas exchange	To evaluate smoking status.	Smoking status of the patients is evaluated.	Improvement in gas exchange.
			To educate patient regarding smoking cessation.	Educate the patient regarding smoking cessation.	
			To educate regarding hazards of smoking.	Patient is educated regarding hazards of smoking.	
			To evaluate current exposures to occupational toxins, indoor and outdoor air pollution.	Current exposures to occupational toxins, indoor and outdoor air pollution is evaluate.	
			To educate the patient regarding indoor and outdoor pollution	Educate the patient regarding indoor and outdoor pollution.	
			To administer broncho-dilators as prescribed.	Administer bronchodilators as prescribed.	
			To instruct and encouage patient in diaphragmatic breathing and coughing.	Instruct and encourage patient in diaphragmatic breathing and coughing.	

Contd...

Contd...

S. No.	Nursing Diagnosis	Objectives	Planning	Implementation	Evaluation
			To demonstrates an exercise plan to be carried out at home.	Demonstrate an exercise plan to the patient which is carried out at home.	
			To educate the patient gradually increase walking time and distance to improve physical condition.	Patient is educated gradually increases walking time and distance to improve physicaly	
			To teach the patient exercise both upper and lower body.	Patient is teach exercise both upper and lower body.	
2.	Atelectasis related to chest infection.	Absence of atelectasis on X-ray and physical examination.	To monitor respiratory status including rate, breath sounds, sings and symptoms of respiratory distress.	Respiratory status is monitor including breath sounds, signs and symptoms of respiratory distress.	Absence of atelectasis on X-ray examination.
			To instruct the patient to encourage diaphragmatic breathing and effective coughing techniques.	Patient is encourage for diaphragmatic breathing and effective coughing technique	
			To promote use of lung expansion techniques, e.g. deep breathing exercise.	Promote use of lung expansion techniques, e.g. deep breathing exercise.	

Contd...

Contd...

S. No.	Nursing Diagnosis	Objectives	Planning	Implementation	Evaluation
3.	Pneumothorax due to infection	Absence of signs and symptoms of pneumothorax	To monitor respiratory status, such as pattern of respiration, breath sounds.	Monitor respiratory status, such as pattern of respiration, breath sounds	Absence of signs and symptoms of pneumothorax
			To assess for chest pain and precipitating factors.	Assessed for chest pain and precipitating factors.	
			To palpate for tracheal deviation/shift away from the affected side.	Palpate for tracheal deviational/shift away from the affected side.	
			To administer analgesic as indicated for chest pain	Analgesic is administer	
4.	Respiratory failure.	Absence of signs and symptoms of respiratory failure.	To monitor respiratory status such as acute respiratory distress.	Respiratory status is monitor, such as acute respiratory distress.	No evidence of respiratory failure on laboratory tests.
			To monitor pulse oximetry and arterial blood gas.	Pulse aximetry and arterial blood gas is monitor every 1 hour.	
			Administer oxygen as indicated mechanical ventilation as prescribed.	Oxygen and mechanical ventilation as administer.	

4. Write short notes on any three:

(a) First aid in insect bite.

(b) Role of nurse in caring of patient with poisoning.

(c) Splinting a leg with fracture.

(d) Emergency care in road accident.

(e) Analgesics.

FIRST AID IN INSECT BITE

- Treat the shock, even in the absence of signs of shock.
- Call the medical assistance in case of known organism—skip this step.
- To remove the stinger on venom sac the traditional advice is to scrape the site with a blade and to avoid pulling with tweezers.
- Remove jewellary from affected limbs in case the limbs swell which would make removal more difficult later.
- If local protocol permits and if the wound is on an extremity place constriction bands above and below the sting or bite site.
- This is done to slow the spread of venom in the lymphatic vessels and superficial veins. The bland should be placed about 2 inch from the wound.
- Keep the limb immobilized and the patient still to prevent distribution of the poison to other parts of the body.

ROLE OF NURSE IN CARING OF PATIENT WITH POISONING

General Management

1. **Collection of history:** A brief but quick history can be taken from the surrounding of the casuality. The history must include.
   a. Any source if known by lookers.
   b. Any clue of the poison
   c. Time of poison
   d. Any sign and symptoms
   e. Method of poison
   f. Amount of poison

   The first aider while taking the history should keep in mind that immediate treatment is necessary as the amount of poison absorbed depend on interval between ingestion and removal of poison. A skillful person will try to take history while he is caring for the patient and will not waste even a single minute.
2. **Identification of poison:** The first step is taking of history can help in the identification of the poison some of the poisons, e.g. the kerosene oil, DDT, etc., so that first aider can identify the poison by smelling the mouth of the patient. These smells can then be correlate with the signs and symptoms appearing in the patient. The identification of the poison helps to carry-out the specific treatment in case of the poison consumed. The specific antidotes available can be used to prevent further complication.
3. **Termination of link with poison:** The first aider has to immediately observe the link and to reduce the contact of patient with poison. Earlier

the termination of the link more easily the patient can be recovered or more easily poison can be removed.

4. **Removal of the poison:** This is an important steps in the management of poisoned patient. The poison can be removed by vomiting gastric lavage or by excretion of poison except some of the poisons the best used method to remove poisons is by vomiting. Vomiting is induced by stimulating pharynx with finger or by giving salty solution gastric lavage is good method of emptying the stomach contents.
5. **Shifting to hospital:** After stabilizing a patient to some extent the patient is then shifted to hospital. Various arrangements are made for shifting as call to ambulance, etc. the patient is then cared under medical supervision.

SPLINTING A LEG WITH FRACTURE

- Immobilize the part.
- Straighten the legs.
- Apply the splints an inner one from the groin to the heel and an outer one from the armpit to the heel tie the splint with the help of bandage.
- Shift the patient to the hospital as soon as possible.

EMERGENCY CARE IN ROAD ACCIDENTS

Emergency Steps

- Look for the presence of any dangerous substance.
- Do not pull casualties form the vehicle that may cause further injuries.
- Call emergency services and if possible disconnect the battery.
- Do not allow anyone to smoke near the vehicle.
- Traffic should be directed 200 meter away from the accidents site with the help of warning trangles.
- Immobilize the car by applying handbrake or placing block under the wheels.
- Look for small children that may be hidden under the seats.

Moving Casualty

- Move the casualty very carefully.
- Immobilize the casualty.
- Enough persons should be present to support all parts of the body and move coordinately.
- Remove in one continuous movement without jerking.

Removal of Trapped Casualty

- Try to move the vehicle away from the casualty first because of danger of fire.
- Mark the exact position of the vehicle and informed to police.

ANALGESICS

- Morphine
- Pethidine
- Pholcodeine
- Dihydrocodeine
- Buprenorphine
- Butorphenol
- Tramadol hydrochloride
- Codeine
- Heroin
- Dextromethorphan
- Pentazocine
- Nalbuphine
- Nalorphine
- Naloxone.

An analgesic is a drug that results in the abolition of sensation of pain. this is different from anesthetic agent, e.g. morphine, which is an analgesics drug makes the patient unable to feel pain but he can still feel the sensation of touch and heat.

5. (a) 1. List two purposes of exercising.

2. List two steps to reduce nosocomial infection in the hospital.
3. List two rich sources of carbohydrates.
4. Write the full form of:
   (i) NPO (ii) Cap
   (iii) IV (iv) SC

(b) Write whether the statements are 'True' or 'False':

1. The normal range of pulse is 100–120/min.
2. Savlon is an antifungal agent.
3. Chest physiotherapy helps to dislodge the secretions in the chest.
4. The eye is cleaned from the outer canthus to the inner canthus.
5. Any systemic infection can raise the body temperature.
6. Sodium hypochlorite solution is effective if it is prepared daily.
7. Cyanosis is a good sign in the assessment of clients progress.

PURPOSE OF EXERCISING

- To stimulate the blood circulation
- To prevent obesity

- To regulate body temperature
- To maintain muscle tone.

TWO STEPS TO REDUCE NOSOCAMIAL INFECTION

- **Disinfection:** The articles used by the patient as well as urine, feces sputum should be properly disinfected.
- **Handwashing:** After handing contaminated articles and patient wash hand properly with soap and water, use mask, gloves and gown also.
- Isolation of infected patient from healthy.

RICH SOURCES OF CARBOHYDRATES

- **Starches:** These are present in cereals (rice, wheat) roots and tubers, potatoes.
- **Cellulose:** This is present in vegetables, fruits and cereals.

WRITE FULL FORM OF

- NPO = Nil per orally
- Cap = Capsule
- IV = Intravenous
- SC = Subcutaneous

WRITE WHETHER THE STATEMENTS ARE 'TRUE' OR 'FALSE'

1. The normal range of pulse is 100 -120/min. **False**
2. Savlon is an antifungal agent. **False**
3. Chest physiotherapy helps to dislodge the secretions in the chest. **True**
4. The eye is cleaned from the outer canthus to the inner canthus. **False**
5. Any systemic infection can raise the body temperature. **True**
6. Sodium hypochlorite solution is effective if it is prepared daily. **True**
7. Cyanosis is a good sign in the assessment of clients progress. **False**

Fundamental of Nursing
November 2009

Time: 3 Hours **Maximum Marks: 75**

Note: *Attempt all questions.*

1. **Define the following terms:** **10×1=10**
   (a) Nurse (b) Pulse
   (c) Auscultation (d) Glossitis
   (e) Infancy (f) Boiling
   (g) Fomites (h) Diuretics
   (i) Intermittent fever (j) Lithotomy position
2. **Write down the purposes of:** **3×5=15**
   (a) Steam inhalation.
   (b) Oral hygiene.
   (c) Air mattress.
3. **You are given the responsibility to take care of a terminally-ill patient:**
   (a) What are the sign and symptoms of a patient approaching death? **5**
   (b) What will you do to meet the needs of the dying patient and his relatives? **10**
   (c) Write down the packing of a dead body with communicable disease. **5**
4. **Write short notes on any three:** **3×5=15**
   (a) Scope of nursing.
   (b) Role of nurse during floods.
   (c) Importance of intake and output recording.
   (d) First-aid of a patient with thermal burns.
   (e) Nurses role in maintaining good nutrition of the patient.

5 **(a)** 1. List two points to be kept in mind while giving foot care to a diabetic patient. **4×2=8**
2. List two factors that promote formation of bedsores.
3. List two purposes of cardiac table.
4. Write the full form of BD and PRN.

(b) Write 'T' if the statement is True and 'F' if the statement is False: **7×1=7**

1. The method of sterilization by using formaldehyde gas is called fumigation.
2. Restrict smoking in the patients unit to prevent accidental fires.
3. Before inserting thermometer in patient's mouth wipe it from stem to bulb.
4. Projectile vomiting is significant of pyloric stenosis and cerebral condition.
5. Potassium permanganate is used as an emollient for mouth care.
6. One purpose of ear irrigation is to remove a grain lodged in ear.
7. Proctoclysis is an evacuation enema.

SOLVED QUESTION PAPER 2009

1. Define the following terms:

(a) Nurse
(b) Pulse
(c) Auscultation
(d) Glossitis
(e) Infancy
(f) Boiling
(g) Fomites
(h) Diuretics
(i) Intermittent fever
(j) Lithotomy position

NURSE

Nurse is a graduate of a recognized nursing school who has met the requirements for a registered nurse in a state in which she is licensed to practice.

PULSE

Pulse is defined as an alternate expansion (rise) and recoil (fall) of an artery as the wave of blood is forced through it during the contraction of left ventricle.

AUSCULTATION

It is the listening to sounds with body with the aid of a stethoscope, fetoscope or directly with the ear placed on the body.

GLOSSITIS

It is defined as inflammation of tongue.

INFANCY

First one year of life is called infancy period.

BOILING

Boling in water for at least 20 minutes kills all germs, boiling for 30 minutes, may kill all spores.

FOMITES

These are articles other than food and drinks, e.g. toys, pencil, pen, clothes, etc., which are infected by patient.

DIURETICS

Which increase the flow of urine.

INTERMITTENT FEVER

The temperature rises from normal or subnormal to high fever and back at regular intervals. The interval may vary from few hours to three days.

LITHOTOMY POSITION

The patient lies on his back with on pillow under the head. The legs are well separated and thigh are well flexed on the abdomen and the legs on the thighs. This position used for the gynecological examination and treatment.

2. Write down the purposes of:

a. Steam inhalation.
b. Oral hygiene.
c. Air mattress.

STEAM INHALATION (PURPOSE)

- To relieve the inflammation of congestion of the mucous membrane of respiratory tract
- To soften the thick and tenacious secretion
- To provide moisture heat and prevent dryness of the mucous membrane of respiratory tract
- To relieve spasm of larynx and bronchi
- To apply antiseptic action by use of menthol. TR Benz co.

ORAL HYGIENE (PURPOSE*)*

- To give freshness to the mouth
- To prevent from infectious
- To increase blood circulation
- To stimulate appetite
- To find out the oral problems
- To prevent from dental carries.

PURPOSES OF AIR MATTRESS

- To prevent bedsore
- To prevent pressure on the body
- To useful for bedridden patient
- To protect from friction.

3. You are given the responsibility to take care of terminally-ill patient.

(a) What are the sign and symptoms of a patient approaching death?

(b) What will you do to meet the needs of the dying patient and his relatives?

(c) Write down the packing of a dead body with communicable disease.

SIGN AND SYMPTOMS OF DEAD PATIENT

- Facial appearance
- Facial muscles relax
- Cheeks become flaccid
- Facial structure changes, so the dentures cannot be worn
- With the dentures removed mouth structure may collapse
- Lips plicker and sink in pucker
- Pale ashy skin
- Sunken eyes
- Sides of the nose drawn in with each inspiration.

Changes in the Sight, Speech and Hearing

- Sight gradually fails
- The pupil fails to react to fight
- Eyes are sunken and half-closed
- Film appears over the eyes
- Speech becomes difficult, confused
- Unintelligent and finally impossible.

Changes in the Respiratory System

- Respiration becomes irregular
- Cheyne stokes rapid and shallow
- Stertorous due to presence of secretion.

Circulatory System

- Circulatory changes cause alteration in the temperature, pulse and respiration
- Radial pulse gradually fails
- Usually pulsations are seen even after the patient has stopped breathing.

Gastrointestinal (GI) System

- Hiccup
- Nausea
- Vomiting
- Abdominal distension
- The gag reflex disappears
- The patient feels the inability to swallow.

Genitourinary System

- Retention of urine
- Distention of bladder
- Incontinence of urine
- Stool due to loss of sphincter control.

Skin and Musculoskeletal System

- The skin becomes pale, cool, sweat
- Ears and nose are cold to touch
- Skin is pale due to congestion of blood in the veins.

Central Nervous System

- Reflexes and pain gradually lost
- Patient may be restless due to lack of oxygen and due to raised body temperature.

Signs of Clinical Death

- Absence of pulse, heart beat, respiration
- Red cell formations stop

- Absense of all reflexes
- Pupils of the eye become fixed and non-reactive to light
- **Rigor mortis:** A stiffening of the body after death is due to fixation of the muscles
- Blue discoloration due to the settling of the blood.

NEEDS OF DYING PATIENT AND THEIR RELATIVES

Psychological Support

There are five psychological stages that dying persons pass through. These are denial, anger, bargaining, depression and acceptance. In these all stages, patient need psychological support and their relatives also because they also suffer from depression and grief.

The psychological needs of dying patient are:

- Relief from loneliness, fear and depression
- Maintenance of security, self-confidence and dignity
- Maintenance of hope
- Meeting the spiritual needs according to his religious customs.

Symptomatic Management

- **Problems associated with breathing:** The dying patient who is restless may be given, the oxygen inhalation to relieve the discomfort. Elevate the head, keep the room well ventilated, keep crowd away.
- **Problems associated with elimination:** Patient needs a care of bowel and bladder. Each problem related to this prevented or a least treated if possible.
- **Problem R/T sense organs:** Patient loses sight, before giving any care touch the patient and say what you are doing. Speak loudly in case of hearing loss.
- **Problems R/T rest and sleep:** All the possible care should be given to reduce pain and to ensure rest and sleep.
- **Problems associated with cleanliness and growing:** Cleanliness and appearance are important until the end cleanliness of skin, hand, mouth, clothing, etc. are to be emphasized.

Care of Dead Patient

- In order to keep the body in normal position and forms, the body should be cared for immediately after death and before rigor mortis occurs.

- The eyes are closed immediately and the body is straightened with the arms laid at sides:
  - Any dentures are removed and mouth is closed.
  - The head elevated on a pillow and a folded towel is used to prop the chin in position. Bandages may be used if necessary.
  - Remove all the appliances used for the care of patient. If N/G tube was in, remove it after aspirating the stomach contents.
  - If O_2 administration remove it.
  - All comfort device removed.
  - If urinary catheter was put in remove it.
  - Remove the ornaments of any type.
  - Send the body as clean and neatly dressed as possible.
  - All orifices are of bodily discharge.
  - Patient chart with all details sent to record section for filling death certificate.

PACKING OF A DEAD BODY WITH COMMUNICABLE DISEASE

Care and packing of a dead body with communicable disease is some like other dead bodies. But same precautions used to prevent. Spreading of communicable disease like.

Terminal Disinfection

After the death of person with communicable disease all the articles, patient room bed, lockers which used by the patient are to be totally disinfectant.

- All the wastage from the dead body properly discard.
- Disinfectant all the articles by using various sterilization methods.
- Handover the body to patients relatives with precaution by telling about disease communicability.

4. Write short notes on any three:

(a) Scope of nursing
(b) Role of nurse during floods
(c) Importance of intake and output recordings
(d) First aid of patient with thermal burns
(e) Nurse role in maintaining good nutrition of patient.

SCOPE OF NURSING

In nursing field, the scope of nursing is very wide. The nursing services are very important part of health care services in the health team. Various opportunities are available for herself personal and professional growth and development, The main areas for her self growth and development are as following.

- Registered nurse-registered midwife (RN-RM) can go for post basic BSc after 2 years clinical experiences
- After BSc in Nursing

  ↓

  MSc Nursing

  ↓

  PhD/M phil and Research
- RN-RM can do various clinical specialization courses in different fields as:
  - Pediatric
  - OT technique
  - Neonatology
  - ICCU
  - ICU
  - Urology
  - Neurology
  - Burn unit
  - Psychiatric nursing, etc.

There are many opportunities available in nursing. These require advanced education leading to varied roles and challenges to nursing personnel. Some expanded nursing roles include nurse practioner clinical nurse, nurse midwife nurse anesthetist, nurse researcher nurse administrator and nurse educator.

In addition to these, professional nurse also functions as a:

- Caregiver
- Decision-maker
- Client advocate
- Manager and coordinator
- Communicator
- Education.

ROLE OF NURSE DURING FLOODS

Flood is natural calamities problem in such situation a large number of people are involved simultaneously. It is difficult to render first aid of so many people at a time. It is necessary to set-up a first aid center at the site of the calamity to all for aid from elsewhere and establish mobile dispensaries.

The responsibilities of the health workers in calamities are as follows:

- To look after the injure and sick persons, providing them with medical and nursing care.
- To prevent spread of communicable diseases.
- To manage the temporary shelter place effectively.
- To look after nutritional requirements of infants and children.
- To manage food and drinking water supply in the center.
- To provide special care to pregnant women, infants old people and patient with chronic disease.
- To give psychological and emotional help to affected people.

IMPORTANCE OF INTAKE AND OUTPUT CHART

- Intake and output chart help the nurse to assess the electrolyte balance of patient.
- It is essential to know the balance between fluid given to patient and secretion from body.
- If intake is more than output it indicates edema and ascities of patient.
- Maintenance of intake and output chart of every patient especially who have renal problem useful to measure the output of patient.
- Maintenance of intake and output chart helpful for records of doctor to plan any nursing intervention.

FIRST AID OF PATIENT WITH THERMAL BURN

- Place the injured part under the slowly running cold water for 10 to 15 minutes.
- If the pain persists then continuously put the water.
- Lie the casualty down and make him comfortable.
- Gently remove any rings, bangles wrist watch, shoes and other constricting clothes.
- Cover the area with clean cloth or dressing.
- Give plenty of fluids to the patient orally.
- Immobalize badly burnt skin.
- Do not use any adhesive dressing and do not apply cotton directly over the area.
- Do not break any blister.
- Do not interfere with any injured area.
- Do not apply lotions, ointments or fat to the injury.
- Dress the area with clean, preferably sterile, non-fluffy material. Arrange for medical care.

NURSE ROLE IN MAINTAINING GOOD NUTRITION OF THE PATIENT

- The diet of every patient in the hospital should be planned according to his need, metabolic changes, food habits and socioeconomic status.
- See that the patient gets the prescribed diet at the proper time. Note whether they take the full quantity of food served for them.
- She should report the quantity of food that is left in the tray.
- Create the environment for the patient room should be well ventilated, quiet, decorated and in order during meals.
- Attractive environment increases the appetite of patient.
- Before offering the food remove all the articles like bedpan, sputum cup, etc.
- Food should be offered according to like and dislike and according to the nutrient requirement of the patient.
- Do not disturb the patient during meal by any painful procedure or by any treatment.
- Place the patient in comfortable position in the bed or out of bed.
- Offer a food to patient in attractive which increase the taste and appetite of patient.
- She provide a meal to the patient who is not able to eat to be orally she provides diet by tube feeding.
- Small and frequent diet given to patient.
- Physical and mental fatigue should be avoided.
- If the nurse sits near the patient and engages in the conversation it makes the meal a pleasure experience for the patient.
- Meals should be served in clean and covered containers.
- Provision should be made to wash hands and the face of the patient before and after the meals.
- The food should be cut into small pieces and have one piece at a time, one food after another.
- The patient should have time to chew and taste the food. Never make hurry to the patient.
- The patient should be encouraged to take a variety of foods.
- Fluid requirement should be met to prevent dehydration.
- The nurse should take every chance to teach the patient and his relative about well balanced diet.

5. (a) 1. List two points to be kept in mind while giving foot care to a diabetic patient.
2. List two factors that promote formation of bedsores.
3. List two purposes of cardiac table.
4. Write the full form of BD and PRN.

POINT KEPT IN MIND WHILE GIVING FOOT CARE TO A DIABETIC PATIENT

- **Patient:** Prevent the foot from friction and pressure advise the patient do not wear ill fitting shoes and socks.
- While cutting nails prevent injuries by cutting straight not round nails.

LIST TWO FACTORS THAT PROMOTE FORMATION OF BEDSORES

- Pressure
- Friction
- Moisture
- Pathogenic microorganism.

Pressure

It is primary cause of pressure sore. The area which comes in contact with mattress are vulnerable area. In this area, blood supply depletion with failure of circulation to weight bearing area resulting in the tissue damage. Causes of pressure are:
- When there are lumps and creases on the bed.
- Incorrect positioning of the body.
- Infrequent change of position.

Moisture

The skin contact with moisture for a period of time can lead to maceration of the skin. Patients who are sweating profusely with incontinence of urine and stools are liable to pressure sores.

LIST TWO PURPOSES OF CARDIAC TABLE

- To maintain the position of cardiac patient
- To help in serving food to the patient.

WRITE THE FULL FORM OF BD AND PRN

BD Bis in Die-Twice a day
PRN Pro-re-Nata-when required.

WRITE 'T' IF THE STATEMENT IS TRUE AND 'F' IF STATEMENT IS FALSE

- The method of sterilization by using formaldehyde gas is called fumigation. **True**

- Restrict smoking in the patients unit to prevent accidental fires. **True**
- Before interesting thermometer in patients mouth wipe it from stem to bulb. **False**
- Projectile vomiting is significant of pyloric stenosis and cerebral condition. **True**
- Potassium permangnate is used as an emollient for mouth care. **False**
- One purpose of ear irrigation is to remove a grain lodged in ear. **True**
- Proctoclysis is an evacuation enema. **True**

Fundamental of Nursing
December 2008

Time: 3 Hours **Maximum Marks: 75**

Note: *Attempt all the questions.*

1. (a) Define nursing.

(b) Discuss the qualities of nurse. **10**

2. (a) Define communication.

(b) List of the barriers of communication. **10**

3. (a) Discuss the importance of documentation in nursing.

(b) List down the type of records used in the ward. **5+5**

4. Elaborate the nursing responsibilities in any two of the following.

(a) Oral medication

(b) Steam inhalation

(c) Mouth care **5+5**

5. Write short notes on:

(a) Health education

(b) First aid in shock. **7½ +7½**

6. Define the following items.

(a) Shock

(b) Hyperpyrexia

(c) Disinfection

(d) Insomnia

(e) Universal precautions

(f) Anoxia

(g) Sitz bath

(h) Fowler's position

(i) Active and passive exercises

(j) Blood pressure **2×10=20**

SOLVED QUESTION PAPER 2008

1. (a) Define nursing.
(b) Discuss the qualities of nurse.

DEFINE NURSING

Ace to ICN

The International Council of Nurses accepted the following definition. "Nursing is the unique function of the nurse that is to assist the individual (sick or well) in the performance of those activities contributing to health or its recovery, that he would perform unaided if he had the necessary strength, will or knowledge".

QUALITIES OF A NURSE

- ***Love for the fellow men:*** She acts and interacts with fellow men.
- ***Honesty and loyalty:*** She shows honesty and loyalty with patients and towards own duty.
- ***Discipline:*** She performs own duty with discipline and follows rules of nursing profession, e.g. simplicity.
- ***Obedience:*** She follows the order of seniors like sister incharge, doctors, etc.
- ***Alertness of intelligent observation:*** She is always alert about patient condition and uses intelligent observations to understand the problems of patients.
- ***Adjustability:*** She is very adjustable in every situation and with limited resources.
- ***Resource:*** *Fullness*—She is able to arrange appropriate interventions for patients.
- ***Economy of time, material and energy:*** She saves time, energy and material by using knowledge, skill and experience.
- ***Courtesy and dignity:*** As a human being she homes a dignity.
- ***Sympathy, empathy:*** She has feelings of sympathy and empathy towards patients.
- ***Common sense:*** She has a common sense to interact with seniors and other persons.
- ***Patience and sense of humor:*** While dealing with patient she show patience and use sense of humor to develop a good improving patient rounds with patient.

- ***Good physical and mental health:*** She is healthy physically as well as mentally.
- *Other qualities:*
  - Generosity
  - Gentleness
  - Ability to inspire confidence
  - Technical competence
  - Tactfulness or poise

2. (a) Define communication.

(b) List of the barriers of communication.

DEFINE COMMUNICATION

Communication can be defined as, the interchange of thoughts or information conveyed to a person or people in such a way that the meaning received is equivalent to that which the initiator of the message intended.

BARRIERS IN COMMUNICATION

A message may be distorted by:

- ***Emotional factors:*** Emotional factors such as fear, suspicion, jealousy, anger, anxiety, grief, prejudices, lack of interest and lack of listening cause disturbances in communication.
- ***Physical factors:*** Some physical problems such as fatigue, illness, speech defects, deafness and pain create problems or disturbances in communication process.
- ***Intellectual factors:*** If a person has low Q, lack of knowledge, and misinterpretation of word then that person feels problem in communication. He is not able to express his own feelings and problems and not able to understand others.
- ***Social factors:*** Difference in cultures, language, race, professional status, socioeconomic status, etc. are the social factors which contribute as a barrier in communication.
- ***Environment at factors:*** Noise, lack of privacy, uncomfortable accommodations, etc. also cause problem in communication.

There are some other barriers which block communication.

- **Changing the subject:** Sudden change in the subject causes loss of interest of people and this loss of interest causes loss of communication.
- **Lack of listening :** If the people do not listen to the topic with attention it fails to get communicated.

- **Inappropriate use of knowledge :** Lack of knowledge about the subject in the to person also causes problems in communication, like:
  - Jumping into conclusions
  - False and inappropriate reassurance
  - Stating one's own opinions and ideas.

3. (a) Discuss the importance of documentation in nursing.

(b) List down the type of records used in the ward.

THE IMPORTANCE OF DOCUMENTATION IN NURSING

- **Communication:** It helps to promote continuity of care among departments throughout twenty four hours of care. It is essential that all personnel provide written documentation of anything they have observed or done with a client to ensure coordination of activities and continuity of care.
- **Quality assurance:** As part of quality assurance program, health care agencies periodically conduct chart audits to determine whether or not the care provided, meets the established standards of client care. So, records are helpful in assuring the quality of care.
- **Legal accountability:** The client's records serve as a legal document of the clients health status and the care received. Properly maintained records help the nurse and protect from legal actions. Nurse and other health care providers cannot remember specific assessments and interventions about a client year after year. Therefore accurate and complete documentation at the time of care is essential.
- **Research:** Nursing and health care research is often carried out by studying client records. The reliability and validity of this research depends on complete and accurate documentation of client data.
- **Diagnostic and therapeutic orders:** It is helpful for nurse to know the diagnosis and therapeutic interventions which were entered in patient records. With the help of this, she is able to provide best possible care to patients.
- **Assessment:** It helps the nurse and other health care personnel agencies to make assessment of the status of the patient.
- **Planning:** After assessment, nurse can plan the nursing care for the patient. Each health care personnel uses the data from the client record to plan care for the client.
- **Education:** Nurses and other members of health team use these records as the educational tools for the patients, their relatives and nursing students.

- **Vital statistics:** Records help in vital statistics and to evaluate the health services.

Others

- Historical document
- Health services planning.

LIST DOWN THE TYPES OF RECORDS USED IN THE WARD

- Outpatient and inpatient records
- Nurse's recording
- Doctor's order sheet
- Graphic charts of temperature, pulse and respiration
- Reports of laboratory examination
- Diet sheet
- Consent form for operations and anesthesia
- Intake and output chart
- Reports of anesthesia, physiotherapy, occupational therapy and other special therapies
- Registers
- Medicolegal cases documentation
- Medication record
- Daily nursing care record
- Progress notes
- Nursing discharge/referral smalls summaries
- Long-term care documentation
- Home care documentation
- Flow sheets.

4. Elaborate the nursing responsibilities in any two of the following.

(a) Oral medication
(b) Steam inhalation
(c) Mouth care.

ORAL MEDICATION

Nursing Responsibility Preliminary Assessment:

- Check the diagnosis and age of the client.
- Check the purpose of medication.
- Check the identification of the clients the name, bed no., etc.
- Check the physician's orders for the correct name of the drug dosage and method of administration.

- Check the nurse's record for the time at which the last dose was given.
- Check the symptoms of over dosage of the drug administered due to the cumulative effect of the drug (e.g. by checking the pulse rate before giving digoxin).
- Check for any contraindication present in the client for an oral intake of the medicine, such as nausea, vomiting, delirium and unconsciousness, negative attitude of the client to the intake of the medicine.
- Check the character of the drugs whether it can be taken safely by the oral method. Some drugs if taken by the mouth will be destroyed by the action of the gastric and intestinal juices, e.g. insulin.
- Check the form of the drug available and correct method of administration.
- Check the presence of oral and esophageal lesions.
- Check the consciousness of the client and ability to follow instruction.
- Check the abilities and limitations in swallowing the medications.
- Check the articles available in the clients unit.

Preparation of the Client

- Explain the procedure to the client
- Assist the client to a sitting position
- Give a mouth wash, if necessary
- If the medication is ill tasting, prepare a drink, e.g. lemon juice
- Protect the bed clothes and garments with a towel placed under the chin across the chest.

After Care of the Client

- Remove the towel and wipe the face with it
- Give comfortable position to patient
- Wash all articles and replace them
- Wash hands
- Record medication given, time, etc.
- Observe the patient for any effect of medicine.

STEAM INHALATION

- Preliminary assessment.
- Check the patient name, bed no. and identification
- Check the diagnosis and the general condition of the patient
- Check the physician order

- Assess the patient's ability for self-care, his ability to move and maintain the desired position
- Assess the level of consciousness and the ability to follow instructions
- Check the articles available in patient unit.

Preparation of the Patient and the Environment

- Explain the procedure to the patient to win his confidence and co-operation. Explain the sequence of the procedure and tell him how he can take the inhalation.
- Make the patient to understand that he has to remain in the bed one to two hours more after the inhalation.
- Ask the patient to go to the toilet for empty the bladder and bowels, if headed.
- For the bedridden patient give bedpan.
- Place the patient in a fowler position with cardiac table in front.
- Close the doors and window and put off the fan to prevent draught.
- Place the sputum cup in a convenient place within the easy reach of the patient.
- Provide a face towel to the patient to wipe the sweating from the face during the inhalation.

After Care of Patients

- Continue the treatment for 15 to 20 minutes
- Remove the inhaler from the patient after the stated time
- Wipe off the perspiration from the face
- Remove the backrest and cardiac table
- Instruct him to remain in bed for 1 to 2 hours to prevent draught
- Take the articles to the utility room
- Record the procedure on the nurses record with date and time
- Return to the patient to assess his comfort and observe any untoward reaction to him, offer hot drinks if needed.

MOUTH CARE

Preliminary Assessment

- Check the condition of the oral cavity
- Check the ability of the client for self-care
- Check the general condition of the client
- The frequently mouth care needed

- Doctor's orders for specific precautions regarding the movement and positioning of the client
- Articles available in client's unit.

Preparation of Client

- Explain the procedure of client to gain the cooperation and confidence of the client.
- Provide privacy.
- Maintain a safe comfortable position for the client.
- If the client is unconscious or completely helpless, turn him to the right side and the nurse stands at the right side of the client to do procedure.
- Place the Mackintosh and face towel across the chest and under the chin to protect the bed clothes and the garments.
- Place the kidney tray close to the cheek with the concave side towards the client or allow the client to adjust the kidney tray to receive the waste.
- Remove dentures and place it in a bowel of clean water.
- Arrange the articles convenient for the nurse and for client.

After Care

- Apply glycerin or any other emollient on the cracked lips and tongue to keep them soft.
- Remove the kidney tray, Mackintosh and towel.
- Make the client comfortable.
- Tidy up the unit.
- Replace all articles at proper place.
- Wash hand.
- Records time and nature of treatment.
- Health teaching to patient about oral hygiene.

5. Write short notes on:

(a) Health education

(b) First aid in shock.

HEALTH EDUCATION

It has been defined as process which effects change in the health practices of people and in the knowledge and attitude related to such changes.

Aims of Health Education

According to WHO

- To ensure that health is valued as an asset in the community.
- To equip the people with skills, knowledge and attitudes to enable them solve their health problems by their own actions and efforts.
- To promote the development and proper use of health services.
- **Areas of health education:** The scope of health education is as wide as community health. In practice, the content of health education may be divided into the following divisions for the sake of simplicity.
- **Human biology:** The structure and functions of the body are always marvel to the laymen. The topic which covered include the structure and functions of the body, how to keep physically fit. The need for exercise, rest and sleep, the effects of alcohol smoking and drugs on the body of first aid.
- **Nutrition:** Education about nutrition has important place against malnutrition. They should be educated about value of nutrients, source, storage, preparation, cooking, serving, eating of food, etc.
- **Hygiene:** Education about hygiene in which includes two tasks personal and environmental hygiene, e.g. bathing, washing hand care of teeth, spitting, coughing, food hygiene, lighting, ventilation, etc.
- **MCH and family planning:** Mothers need to be taught about balanced diets, baby care, infant feeding, weaning and immunization, family planning.
- **Prevention of communicable diseases:** Information is given about mode of spread of common communicable disease and protection by immunization against these disease.
- **Prevention of accidents:** Accidents occur in there main areas–the home, the road and work place, safety education should be directed to these areas.
- **Use of health service:** One of the declared aims of health education is to make educated people best use of health services.
- **Mental health:** It is also special areas which needing health education.
- **Principles of health education:** Interest, it is very important because without interest people will not learn. The Health education must be based on the health needs of the people.
- **Participation:** Participation of people is helpful in learning, because personal participation increase personal acceptance.

- **Comprehension:** In health education, we must know the level of understanding education and literacy of the people and mental capacity of the people.
- **Motivation:** Motivation is very important for education we try to motivate individuals and groups to accept new ideas.
- **Reinforcement:** Reinforcement should be given to people help to make the learning permanent.
- **Good human relationship**: The health educator must be kind and sympathetic. People must accept him as their real friend.

FIRST AID IN SHOCK

Shock is defined as inadequate tissue perfusion. It is used by various disorders that result in decreased oxygenation at the cellular level.

Shock is commonly discussed under three types:

1. Hypovolemic shock
2. Cardiogenic shock
3. Distributive shock.

First aid for Hypovolemic Shock

- Lie down the patient on the floor
- Give psychological support to the patient and family
- Check the skin turgor of the patient by pinching and see whether the skin goes back to its original position within 1 second or not
- Loosen the clothes of the patient
- Lower the head and raise foot end
- If there is any bleeding, stop the bleeding by pressing or wrap any bandage or any cloth
- Shift the patient to the hospital as soon as possible.

First aid for Distributive Shock

- Place person in a head down.
- Reassure the patient and family.
- Clean the mouth of patient with clean cloth.
- Check the respiration of the patient.
- Maintain the TP of patient.
- Shift the patient to hospital as soon as possible.

First aid for Cardiogenic Shock

- Observe the patient closely for signs and symptoms of shock.
- Give position to the patient, including elevating the legs, elevating the head, leaving the trunk flat, shoulder slightly.
- Check the respiration of the patient.
- Ventilate the room by opening the doors and window.
- Clean the mouth of the patient if there is any secretions in the mouth.
- Tilt the head toward outside, so that the patient does not aspirate the secretions.
- To maintain the normal respiratory rate 24/min is needed for mouth to mouth respiration in emergency.
- If there is any bleeding cardiac shock due to bleeding then press the bleeding area, so that to restore the blood volume.
- Do cardiopulmonary resuscitation CPR to the patient, so that the patient gain its cardiac functioning.
- Shift the patient to the hospital as soon as possible.

6. Define the following items.

(a) Shock
(b) Hyperpyrexia
(c) Disinfection
(d) Insomnia
(e) Universal precautions
(f) Anoxia
(g) Sitz bath
(h) Fowler's position
(i) Active and passive exercises
(j) Blood pressure.

SHOCK

Shock is defined as inadequate tissue perfusion. Inadequate tissue perfusion can be caused by various disorders that result in decreased oxygenation at the cellular level.

HYPERPYREXIA

Temperature above 105° F is called hyperpyrexia.

DISINFECTION

It means destroying of all the pathogenic organisms.

INSOMNIA

It is defined as the inability to sleep or it is a lessening of the duration or depth of sleep.

UNIVERSAL PRECAUTIONS

It is isolation technique intended to confine the microorganisms within a given and recognized area. There are number of isolation techniques and precautions used to prevent spread of infection.

ANOXIA

It is the lack of oxygen in the tissues.

SITZ BATH

It is a bath, which is taken in a sitting position sitz is a German word means seat.

FOWLER'S POSITION

This is a more erect position in which an effort is made to maintain the position of the patient in sitting posture as nearly upright as possible.

ACTIVE AND PASSIVE EXERCISE

- **Active exercise:** Active exercise is the type of physical activity performed by the patient without assistance.
- **Passive exercise:** A passive exercise the movement or activity is carried out by the help of other person.

BLOOD PRESSURE

Blood pressure is the force exerted by the blood against the walls of the blood vessels as it flows through them. Normal BP of healthy individual is 120/80 mm Hg.

Fundamental of Nursing
October 2007

Time: 3 Hours | **Maximum Marks: 75**

Note: *Attempt all Questions:*

1. **Define the following terms:** **10 × 1 = 10**
   (a) Hyperpyrexia
   (b) Dyspnea
   (c) Autoclaving
   (d) Glossitis
   (e) Bedsore
   (f) Barrier nursing
   (g) Shock
   (h) Anoxia
   (i) Cyanosis
   (j) Pulse
2. **Write short notes on any four of the following:** **4 × 5 = 20**
   (a) Decubitus ulcer
   (b) Functions of hospital
   (c) First aid of burn case
   (d) Importance of personal hygiene
   (e) Sterilization of glass syringes
   (f) Contraindication of oral medication
3. **Write down the purpose of the following:** **5 × 3 = 15**
   (a) Purposes of giving hot water bottle
   (b) Purposes of steam inhalation
   (c) Puroposes of admission bed
4. **Write down the nursing responsibilities of the following:** **5 × 4 = 20**
   (a) Prevention of bedsores
   (b) Patient with constipation
   (c) For giving cold applications to the patient
   (d) A patient having diarrhea

5. Put 'F' if the statement is false and put 'T' if the statement is true, in the given space. **10 × 1 = 10**

- Before inserting thermometer in patient mouth, it should be wiped from bulb to stem.
- After giving back care, methylated spirit is applied as it is a best cleansing agent.
- When body temperature is below 30°C. It is termed as pyrexia.
- Clinical thermometer should be washed with hot water after use.
- Pulse deficit is the term used when there is difference in apical pulse and the radial pulse.
- While giving enema, enema can should be hanged at 45 cm height from patient's body.
- Water hammer pulse is not a sign of shock.
- Determination of the nature and extent of disease, is also termed as diagnosis.
- Symptomatology is the study of signs and symptoms of disease.
- Auscultation is not a method of assessment.

SOLVED QUESTION PAPER 2007

1. Define the following terms:

(a) Hyperpyrexia
(b) Dyspnea
(c) Autoclaving
(d) Glossitis
(e) Bedsore
(f) Barrier nursing
(g) Shock
(h) Anoxia
(i) Cyanosis
(j) Pulse

HYPERPYREXIA

The temperature above 105°F is called hyperpyrexia.

DYSPNEA

It is defined as difficult or labored breathing.

AUTOCLAVING

It is the process of sterilization of articles by steam under pressure using an apparatus called autoclave.

GLOSSITIS

It is defined as inflammation of the tongue.

BEDSORE

It is defined as the ulcerated or sloughed area of tissues subjected to pressure from lying on mattress or sitting on a chair for a prolonged period of time resulting is the slowing of circulation and finally death of tissues. It is also known as pressure sore or decubitus ulcer.

BARRIER NURSING

Barrier nursing or isolation technique is intended to confine the microorganisms within a given and recognized area. There are a number of isolation techniques and precautions used in prevention of spread of infection, e.g. respiratory isolation, enteric isolation, wound and skin isolation, etc.

SHOCK

It is defined as an inadequate tissue perfusion can be caused by various disorders that result in decreased O_2 at the cellular level. It occurs due to loss of blood, fluid from the body, etc.

ANOXIA

It is the lack of oxygen in the tissues.

CYANOSIS

It is defined as the blueness or discoloration of the skin and mucous membrane caused by lack of oxygen in the tissues.

PULSE

Pulse is defined as an alternate expansion (rise) and recoil (fall) of an artery as the wave of blood is forced through it during the contraction of left ventricle.

2. **Write short notes on any four of the following:**
   (a) Decubitus ulcer
   (b) Functions of hospital
   (c) First aid of burn case
   (d) Importance of personal hygiene
   (e) Sterilization of glass syringes
   (f) Contraindication of oral medication

DECUBITUS ULCER (BEDSORE)

Decubitus ulcer is also known as pressure sore or decubiti are ulcerated of tissue subjected to pressure from lying on mattress or sitting on a chair for a prolonged period of time resulting in the slowing of circulation and finally death of tissue.

Causes of Pressure Sores

1. **Direct of immediate causes:**
   - **Pressure:** It is considered to be the primary of bedsore. The areas of tissue against the mattress are vulnerable areas. The pressure in these areas causes depletion of blood supply with the failure of circulation to the weight bearing area resulting to tissue damage. The reasons of pressure are.
     - When there are lumps on the bed
     - Incorrect positioning of the body
     - Infrequent change of position
   - **Friction:** Friction of the skin with a rough or hard surface can cause tissue damage. Contact with the rough surface of the bed, wrinkles on the bed clothes, hard surface of the plaster casts at splints, foreign bodies on the bed, careless handling of bedpan, pulling sheet under the patient, etc. are causes of friction.
   - **Moisture:** The skin contact with moisture for long times also cause bedsore. Excessive sweating and micturition of urine on bed is causes moisture and makes person prone to pressure sore.
   - **Presence of pathogenic organism:** Lack of cleanliness harbors pathogenic organism and infection settles on the skin causing pressure sores.
2. **Predisposing causes:**
   - Impaired circulation
   - Lowered vitality
   - Very thin

- Edema
- Obesity.

Common sites:

- One the area that bear weight
- It happens more be on body prominences of the body where less blood supply
- Thin layer of skin.

The other common sites depend upon the position of the patient.

In supine position:

- Back of the head
- Scapula
- Sacral region
- Elbow and heels.

In side-lying position:

- Ears
- Acromion process of shoulders
- Ribs
- Greater trochanter of lip
- Medial and lateral condyles of knees
- Malleolus of the ankle joint.

In prone position:

- Ears
- Cheek
- Acromion process
- Breasts
- Genitalia (male)
- Knees and toes.

Patients Susceptible to Pressure Sores

- Actually ill patients
- Bedridden elderly patient
- Obese patient
- Very thin patient
- Patient under sedation
- Paralyzed patients
- Neurologic patient with lack of sensation
- Edematous patients
- Malnourished patient with lack of protein and vitamins
- Patient with complete bedrest

- Surgical patient with limited movements
- Patient with excessive body discharges or drainage from wounds
- Diabetic patients
- Patient with profuse sweating and incontinence of urine and stool.

Sign/Symptoms of Pressure Sore

The sign/symptoms include:

- Redness
- Tenderness
- Discomfort
- The area becomes cold to touch and insensitive
- There is local edema
- Later the area becomes blue, purple
- Due to continued pressure
- The circulation is cut off.

Prevention of Pressure Sore

- Identification of patients who are particularly prone to develop of bed-sore.
- Daily examination of patient of redness discoloration, etc.
- Keep the patient clean and dry.
- Change the position of patient every two hours.
- Use bed cradle to lift off the weight of bed linen.
- Keep the patient's skin well lubricated to prevent cracking by using powder.
- Protect the damaged skin.
- Provide the patient with adequate fluids and with a nourishing diet that is high in protein and vitamins.
- Attend to the pressure points to stimulate the circulation.
- Change the position every two hourly or frequently.
- Call assistance and lift the patient before giving and taking bedpans.
- Provide a smooth, firm, wrinkle free bed to patient.
- Use special matters and other comfort device.
- Change the linen as soon as they become wet.
- Teach the patient and their relatives about hygienic care of the skin.

Treatment of Decubitus Ulcer

The decubitus ulcer once occurs is difficult to treat. The nurse should remember that the pressure sores are prone to infection.

The following steps are taken by the nurses:

- Report to the sister incharge and the physician the early symptom of a bedsore, so that steps may be taken as early as possible to prevent further damage.
- Whenever possible, take off the pressure from the decubitus ulcers by placing the patient on pillows or foam cushion or change the position of the patient.
- Prevent the ulcerated area from becoming infected. Follow strict aseptic technique.
- A cleaning agent is used to clean the ulcerated area, e.g. normal saline.
- Apply all the possible measures for the healing of the wound.
- Application of waterproof ointment, e.g. zinc oxide on the surface of the wound will prevent infection of the underlying tissues.
- If infection is settled, it may be necessary to give some of the antibiotics prescribed by the physician.

FUNCTIONS OF HOSPITAL

A hospital is an integral part of a social and medical organization. The function of which is to provide for the population the complete health care, both curative and preventive. The hospital is also a center for the training of health workers and for research.

The functions of the hospital are:

- Care of the sick and injured
- Prevention of disease and promotion of health
- Diagnosis and treatment of disease
- Medical education
- Research.

FIRST AID OF BURN CASE

Injuries that result from direct exposure to any thermal, chemical, electrical and radiation source are termed burn.

First Aid Measures

- Put out the fire, with water or wrapping in a blanket.
- Do not allow the person on fire to sun especially into the fresh air.
- Immerse the burnt part in cold water, keep the part in cold water for 15 to 20 minutes. If that is not possible, soak clean both in cold water and put it over the burnt area.

- If water is not available, cover burnt area with sterile dressing.
- Avoid exposure to air.
- In case of face burn, make the dressing in the shape of a mask, with holes at the level of the nose for breathing.
- Remove rings, bracelets, shoes and any other tight fitting articles, as swelling may develop later on, making it difficult to remove them.
- Cover large burnt area with clean linen.
- Arrange for immediate transfer to a hospital.
- When a large area is damaged, pack, ice in a towel and apply it to the burnt area during transfer to a hospital.
- Do not put flour butter or baking soda on the burn.
- Do not put lotion, ointments or oil on burnt area.
- Do not prick or break any blister that may form.
- Do not handle or touch the patient more than absolutely necessary.
- Do not remove adhering particles of clothing.

In chemical burn:

- Remove the contaminated clothing carefully after soaking it in water.
- Flood the affected area with cold water, wash thoroughly.
- Give general treatment for burns.

In sunburn:

- Remove the patient into shade.
- Cool the affected area with cold compresses.
- Give non-alcoholic cold drinks.
- Give general treatment for burn, call a doctor.

IMPORTANCE OF PERSONAL HYGIENE

Define Personal Hygiene

Personal hygiene refers to maintenance of cleanliness of our body.

Importance

This is very important for our body to keep us healthy. In order to maintain ourselves physically, mentally and socially healthy, personal hygiene is very important. The importance of maintaining personal hygiene is as follows:

- To clean our body off from dirt and bacteria
- To keep the body protected from infection
- To provide an aesthetic sense
- To keep us fresh and cheerful look

- It increases confidence and mental status
- To prevent us from illness
- To keep the body free from bad odor.

So maintenance of personal hygiene gives fresh look and helps to concentrate on work.

STERILIZATION OF GLASS SYRINGES

- Syringes make an expensive and common item of the glassware used in the hospital.
- Rinsing immediately after use is important to prevent the pistons sticking to the barrels.
- Stock syringes may be placed in 25% aqueous solution of glycerin and boiled for 10 minutes.
- If the needle is stuck to the hub of the syringe, immersing it in the boiling water will make the metal expand and separate them.
- When cleaning and sterilizing syringes, the barrels and pistons number should be kept together to avoid wasting time later in matching the parts.
- Sterilization by hot air is the best method of sterilization for glass syringes.
- Steam or chemical sterilization is more effective.
- If the syringes are boiled in distilled water silicate is taken from the glass and result in a slow deterioration of the syringes.
- Never put the glass in boiling water.
- Put the glassware in cold water and bring to the boiling point.

CONTRAINDICATION OF ORAL MEDICATION

Definition

Administration of medication by mouth

Contraindications

- Alteration in GI tract like vomiting
- Reduced GI motility
- Surgical removal of a portion of the GI tract
- Inability to swallow
- Patient with neuromuscular disorders
- Patient with mouth lesions

- Patients with gastric aspiration
- Before certain tests/surgery
- Unconscious or confused patients
- Patients who are on NPO status
- Patients with poor gag reflex.

3. Write down the purpose of the following:

(a) Purposes of giving hot water bottle

(b) Purposes of steam inhalation

(c) Puroposes of admission bed

PURPOSES OF GIVING HOT WATER BOTTLE

- To stimulate circulation
- To promote suppuration
- To promote healing
- To relieve pain
- To reduce inflammation and congestion
- To supply warmth and comfort
- To relieve muscle spasm
- To relieve retention of urine.

PURPOSES OF STEAM INHALATION

- To reduce the inflammation and congestion of mucous membrane of respiratory tract
- To soften thick mucus and help it expulsion from respiratory tract, this is to relieve cough
- To provide heat and moisture to prevent dryness of mucous membrane of lungs and upper respiratory passage after operation, e.g. tracheostomy
- To relieve spasm of larynx and bronchi
- To provide antiseptic action to the respiratory passage by using medications as ordered.

PURPOSES OF ADMISSION BED

- Admission bed is prepared for a new admission patient
- To clean the patient
- To observe the patient from heat to toe
- To provide comfort to the patient
- To help the physician to do the physical examination.

4. Write down the nursing responsibilities of the following:
(a) Prevention of bedsores
(b) Patient with constipation
(c) For giving cold application to the patient
(d) A patient having diarrhea.

PREVENTION OF BEDSORES

Refer Paper 2007, Q. No.2 (a).

PATIENT WITH CONSTIPATION

Constipation is the difficult evacuation of hard stool requiring much use of a supportive muscles.

Prevention and Management of Constipation

- **Health teaching:** Health education to patient who are suffering from constipation about cause of constipation and factors affecting it.
- **Adequate intake of diet:** Educate the patient to take adequate amount of diet, because inadequate intake of diet or too little diet may not stimulate the peristalsis movement.
- **Intake of roughage in diet:** Education to patient to take foods which containing high fibrous content. Such as raw and cooked vegetables, fruits, whole grain, cereals, etc.
- **Establishing a habit pattern:** Educate the patient to develop a habit to sit on the toilet daily.
- **Relaxation:** Provide relaxed environment to patient because tension, worry, anger, hurry, fear, etc. interfere with defecation reflex.
- **Privacy:** Arrange privacy for patient during defecation leaving the patient alone and providing him privacy with curtains, etc.
- **Posture:** A squatting position is most effective posture during defecation because the individual can increase the intra-abdominal pressure, necessary for expelling the feces.
- **Exercise:** Advise the patient for exercise which helps to improve muscle tone.
- **Adequate amount of fluid intake:** Normally an individual should take 2000 to 3000 mL of fluid in 24 hours.
- **Use of laxatives, suppositories and enemas:** Use of these should be avoided as much as possible because they are habit forming but when all preventive measures fail then it is used to relieve constipation.

FOR GIVING COLD APPLICATION TO THE PATIENT

- Assess the condition of the patient prior to, during and after the application of the cold therapy.
- Maintain the correct temperature for the entire duration of the application.
- Never use any equipment unless you understand its operation completely.
- There must be recovery period between the applications as continuous application of heat or cold can harm tissues.
- Expose the patient only to a safe temperature.
- Never ignore the complaints of a patient however small they appear to be.
- The patient should not be left alone even for a short period of time.
- Squeeze off excess of water.
- When patient has loss of sensation or unconscious used cold application carefully.
- Find out any cause of complication early.
- After procedure drying the part gently by patting not by rubbing.
- Protect the patient from getting chills.
- In hyperpyrexia, the temperature of the body should be brought down gradually and steadily. Sudden cooling is dangerous to the patient.

NURSING CARE OF PATIENT WITH DIARRHEA

Replacement of Fluid and Electrolytes

The fluid lost from the body should be replaced, when oral fluids, may be given plenty of oral fluids:

- If nausea, vomiting also present and if there is marked dehydration, the fluids are given by the IV route
- Potassium losses may be great with diarrhea and therefore, food and fluids containing potassium should be encouraged.
- Small frequent feedings of bland food may be helpful to meet the nutritional needs of the patient avoid food containing chillies, spice, excessively hot and cold food, etc.
  - Make arrangement for use of a bedpan of commode, which is placed in convenient and accessible place.
  - **Care of skin:** Care of skin is essential specially the anal region. It can be prevented by proper clearing and drying of the area after each defecation.

- **Adequate rest:** Provide adequate rest to patient to reducing the physical activity is helpful is lessening the bowel activity.
- **Psychological support:** If the cause of diarrhea is sustained anxiety patient should be reassured.
- **Medication:** The usual medications which are administered to the patient in diarrhea are antidiarrheal, demulcents, astringents, antiseptics, sedatives and anti-spasmodic should be given.

5. Put 'F' if the statement is false and put 'T' if the statement is true, in the given space.

Ans.
- Before inserting thermometer in patient mouth, it should be wiped from bulb to stem. **True**
- After giving back care, methylated spirit is applied as it is a best cleansing agent. **False**
- When body temperature is below 30°C. It is termed as pyrexia. **False**
- Clinical thermometer should be washed with hot water after use. **False**
- Pulse deficit is the term used when there is difference in apical pulse and the radial pulse. **True**
- While giving enema, enema should be hanged at 45 cm height from patient's body. **True**
- Water hammer pulse is not a sign of shock. **False**
- Determination of the nature and extent of disease, is also termed as diagnosis. **True**
- Symptomatology is the study of signs and symptoms of disease. **True**
- Auscultation is not a method of assessment. **False**

Fundamental of Nursing
September 2006

Time: 3 Hours **Maximum Marks: 75**

Note: *Attempt all the questions and their parts in continuity*

1. Define the following terms: **1×10=10**

(a) Dyspnea (b) Temperature
(c) Auditor (d) Isolation
(e) Conduction (f) Autoclaving
(g) Osmosis (h) Dysuria
(i) Hearing aid (j) Asepsis

2. (a) Define pulse. **2**

(b) Enlist various sites to feel pulse. **3**

(c) Explain factors affecting pulse rate. **5**

3. (a) Give classification of enema. **5**

(b) Write down stepwise procedure for giving soap and water enema along with scientific principles. **5**

4. Write down the following: **2×5=10**

(a) Care of rubber goods.
(b) Contraindications of oral temperature.
(c) Properties of true solution.
(d) Observations of urine.
(e) Type of abnormal respiration.

5. (a) Discuss qualities of good nurse. **5**

(b) Write nursing care in diarrhea. **5**

(c) Explain nursing care of dysphonic patient. **5**

6. Write short notes on any four of the following: **5×4=20**

(a) Snake bite
(b) Records and reports
(c) Heat transmission
(d) O_2 administration
(e) Importance of first aid

SOLVED PAPER SEPTEMBER 2006

1. Define the following terms:

(a) Dyspnea
(b) Temperature
(c) Auditor
(d) Isolation
(e) Conduction
(f) Autoclaving
(g) Osmosis
(h) Dysuria
(i) Hearing aid
(j) Asepsis

DYSPNEA

It is defined as difficulty in breathing.

TEMPERATURE

It is balance between heat loss and heat produced by the body.

AUDITORY

It is sense of hearing.

ISOLATION

It means separation of infected person to healthy person to prevent spreading of disease from one to another person.

CONDUCTION

It is the transfer of heat directly through a substance from hot part to the cold part from one molecule to the other. Very little heat is lost by conduction.

AUTOCLAVING

It is the process of sterilization of articles by steam under pressure using an apparatus called autoclave.

OSMOSIS

The passage of fluid from a low to higher concentration through a semipermeable membrane.

DYSURIA

It is a painful micturition.

HEARING AID

An apparatus used by those with impaired hearing for amplifying sound.

ASEPSIS

Freedom from infection or prevention of contact with microorganisms.

2. (a) Define pulse.

(b) Enlist various sites to feel pulse.

(c) Explain factors affecting pulse rate.

DEFINE PULSE

It is an alternate expansion (rise) and fall (recoil) of an artery as the wave of blood is forced through it during the contraction of the left ventricle.

SITES TO FEEL PULSE

- Radial artery in front of wrist
- Temporal artery over temporal bone
- Carotid artery at the side of neck
- Brachial artery above elbow
- Femoral artery in the groin
- Popliteal artery in back of the knee
- The dorsalis pedis artery on the foot
- The posterior or tibial artery behind the medial malleolus
- Apical pulse palpated direct from heart.

THE FACTORS AFFECTING PULSE RATE

Age

The very young have a rapid pulse rate. The adults have normal range of 60 to 100 per minute. The very old have slow pulse rate.

Sex

The female has a high pulse rate than male.

Physique

The short person with small body built has more rapid pulse rate than the tall heavy individual.

Exercise

Increased muscular activity increases pulse rate.

Food

Indigestion food causes a slight in the pulse rate for several hours.

Posture

Pulse rate is rapid in standing position than sitting and lying position.

Emotion

Mental and emotional disturbance increase pulse rate.

Application of Heat

Application of heat can increase pulse rate.

Pain

Pain increases pulse rate.

Increased Body Temperature

When the body temperature raises the pulse rate tends to raise.

Disease Condition

Loss of blood, injury, shock increase the pulse rate. In typhoid fever the pulse rate tends to slow.

Drugs

Stimulant drugs, e.g. caffeine, atropine, adrenaline, etc. will raise the pulse rate. Sedative drugs can reduce the pulse rate.

Cold Application

Cold application can reduce pulse rate.

3. (a) Give classification of enema.
(b) Write down stepwise procedure for giving soap and water enema along with scientific principles.

CLASSIFICATION OF ENEMA

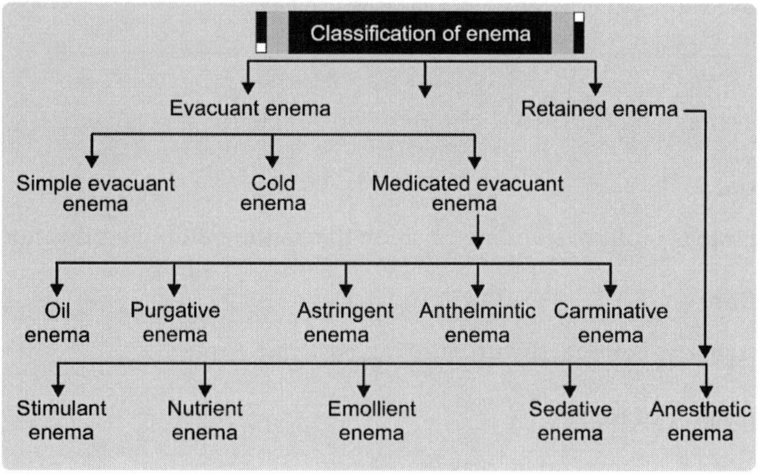

STEPS OF PROCEDURE WITH PRINCIPLES

S. No.	Steps of Procedure	Principles
1.	Wash hands	To prevent cross infection.
2.	Attach the tubing to the enema can and clamp the tube.	To prevent the solution and be ready for the administration.
3.	Prepare the solution at the required temperature. Add 30 mL of soap jelly to 600 mL of water severe. Test the temperature of solution at the inner aspect of the wrist. Remove the form can.	Temperature above 43°C may injure tissues and temperature below 21°C may produce cramping.
4.	Hang the can with the solution on the stand and adjust the height at 45 cm from the anus.	The rate and flow increase according to height of can.
5.	Attach a rectal tube to the tubing loosen the screw clamp and let a small amount of fluid to run into the kidney tray.	Running the fluid through tube will help to expel air form the tubing. Regulate the flow of the solution by adjusting the screw clamp.
6.	Lubricate the tip of the rectal tube about 2 to 4 inches from the tip.	Lubrication will prevent friction.
7.	Lubrication is applied to piece	To prevent the blockage of tube.
8.	Separate the patient's buttock to visualize the anus clearly and insert the tip 8 to 10 cm. gently while the patient exhales deep breath.	Forceful insertion of the rectal tube may injure the anal or rectal tissue.

9.	During the administration of the fluid ask the patient to take breaths.	Breathing with open mouth relaxes the abdominal muscles.
10.	Temporarily stop the administration of the solution if patient has an urge to defecate.	Temporary stoppage of the fluid will relax the bowels as peristaltic movement is passed off.
11.	Continue the fluid administration to give about 500 to 1000 mL of solution stop the procedure if the patient develops discomfort.	
12.	Clamp the tubing, gently remove by pulling it through 3 to 4 layers of rag piece.	Holding the rag pieces around the tube cleanses the tube by removing the feces from the tube.
13.	Discard the rag pieces in the paper bag. Detect the rectal tube and place it in the kidney tray.	Avoid contamination of the articles and environment with the solid articles.

4. Write down the following:

(a) Care of rubber goods.
(b) Contraindications of oral temperature.
(c) Properties of true solution.
(d) Observations of urine.
(e) Type of abnormal respiration.

CARE OF RUBBER GOODS

The rubber goods in common use are air cushion, Mackintoshes, hot water, bottles, ice caps, ice collars, rubber tube, catheters, rectal tubes, glove and rubber beds.

- The nurses should make all efforts to prolong the like of the rubber goods.
- They should be purchased only after their nature and durability have been investigated.
- They should not be exposed to excessive chemical, light, heat or moisture because long time contact with these agents damage the articles.
- They should not be folded.
- Never use any pin to fix the rubber goods anywhere.
- Never use any sunlight.
- Rubber goods should never dried by direct heat.
- Any fluid split on them should be wiped off at once.
- When storing care must be taken, so that no two surfaces come in contact with each other.
- They should not be tied in knots.

- They should not be hung on hooks or nails.
- Clean the all rubber good before storing.
- Do not store wet rubber good because they stick to each other and torn.

CONTRAINDICATION OF ORAL TEMPERATURE

- Patients who are extremely nervous, delirious, unconscious, hysterical and mentally confused and those who cannot follow instructions.
- The patient having convulsions.
- Mouth breather.
- Patients who have injuries, inflammations or operations of mouth.
- Extremely week persons who are not able to hold the thermometer under the tongue.
- Persons suffering from frequent attack of cough.
- Children under six years of age.
- Immediately after taking hot or cold drink, cigarette, smoking, chewing gum or betal leaves the temperature should not be taken by mouth.

PROPERTIES OF TRUE SOLUTION

- **Size of particles:** The size of solute particles is less than one manometer.
- **Visibility:** The solute particles are invisible by naked eye.
- **Separation:** The solute and solvent cannot be separated by ordinary filtering or ultra filtration.
- **Settling:** The solute particles do not settle.
- **Brownian movement:** Do not show Brownian movements.
- **Tidal effect:** Do not show tidal effect.

OBSERVATION OF URINE

- **Volumes:** 1000 to 2000 mL of urine is excreted in 24 hours. It increases in cold and decreases in hot weather.
- **Appearance:** The normal urine is clear with no deposit.
- **Odor:** The normal urine has an aromatic odor.
- **Reaction:** Reaction of the normal urine is slightly acidic.
- **Specific gravity:** The specific gravity of urine varies from 1:016 to 1:025, with normal fluid intake.
- **Constituents of the urine:**
  - Water 96%
  - Urea 2%
  - Uric acid 2% and other constituents, creatinine, phosphates, oxalates.

Observation of Urine in Disease

- **Volume:**
  - Sometimes increase is known as polyuria
  - Sometimes decrease is known as oliguria
  - Sometimes total absent is anuria
  - Failure of kidney to secrete urine is suppression.
- **Color:**
  - Green or brownish yellow (Bile salts of bile pigments)
  - Reddish brown (urobilinogen)
  - Bright red (A large amount of fresh blood)
  - Pink (Small amount of fresh blood)
  - Smoky brown (Blood pigments)
  - Milky white (Chyluria in filariases)
- **Odor:** Sweetish or fruity odor is due to the presence of ketone bodies.
- **Appearance:** Cloudy appearance is due to the presence of phosphates:
  - **Mucus:** Appear flocculent cloud
  - **Pus:** Settles as heavy cloud
  - **Stones:** As fine sand
  - **Uric acid:** As grains of pepper.
  - **Reaction:** Alkaline reaction.
  - **Specific gravity:** 1.001 to 1.60.

Constituents

- Albuminuria in kidney damage
- Acetone glycosuria in diabetes
- **Bile:** Obstructive jaundice.

TYPE OF ABNORMAL RESPIRATION

- **Tachypnea (Polypnea):** It is an increased respiratory rate over 24 breaths per minute.
- **Bradypnea:** It is a decreased respiratory rate less than 10 breaths per minute.
- **Apnea:** Total cessation of breathing. This may be periodic as seen in Cheyne-Stokes respiration.
- **Hyperpnea:** It is an increase in the depth of respiration.
- **Orthopnea:** The patient can breath only in upright position.
- **Stertorous respiration:** It is a noisy breathing snoring sounds are made by air passage through the secretions as seen in acute alcoholism.

- **Stridor:** A harsh, vibrating, shrill sound produced during respiration as seen in upper airway obstruction.
- **Rale:** An abnormal ratting or bubling sound caused by the mucus in the airway.
- **Wheeze:** The high pitched, musical whistling sound that occurs with the partial obstruction of smaller bronchi and bronchioles.
- **Sigh:** A very deep inspiration followed by a prolonged expiration.
- **Air hunger:** A form of dyspnea in which there are deep sighing respiration.
- **Cheyne-stokes respiration:** It consists of a series of respirations that gradually become deeper and noises until a climax is reached.
- **Disphonia:** Difficulty in breathing.
- **Cyanosis:** Bluish or discoloration of the skin or mucous membrane caused by lack of oxygen in the tissues.
- **Anoxia:** It is lack of oxygen in the tissue.
- **Anoxemia hypoxemia:** It is the lack of oxygen in the bloodstream
- **Asphyxia:** It is the state of suffocation.

5. (a) Discuss qualities of good nurse.
(b) Write nursing care in diarrhea.
(c) Explain nursing care of dysphonic patient.

QUALITIES OF A NURSE ARE AS FOLLOWS

- Love for the fellow men
- Honesty and loyalty
- Discipline and obedience
- Alertness and intelligent observation
- Technical competence
- Dependability and adjustability
- Ability to inspire confidence
- Resourcefulness, economy of time, material and energy
- Courtesy and adjustability, dignity
- Sympathy, empathy, tact and poise
- Intelligence and common sense
- Patience and sense of humor
- Good physical and mental health
- Generosity
- Gentleness and quietness.

NURSING CARE OF PATIENT WITH DIARRHEA

Replacement of Fluid and Electrolytes

The fluid lost from the body should be replaced, when oral fluids, may be given plenty of oral fluids:

- If nausea, vomiting also present and if there is marked dehydration, the fluids are given by the IV route.
- Potassium losses may be great with diarrhea and therefore food and fluids containing potassium should be encouraged.
- Small frequent feedings of bland food may be helpful to meet the nutritional need of the patient avoid food containing chillies, spice, excessively hot and cold food, etc.
- Make arrangement for use of a bedpan of commode which is placed in convenient and accessible place.
- **Care of skin:** Care of skin is essential specially the anal region. It can be prevented by proper cleaning and drying of the area after each defecation.
- **Adequate rest:** Provide adequate rest to patient to reducing the physical activity is helpful is lessening the bowel activity.
- **Psychological support:** If the cause of diarrhea is sustained anxiety patient should be reassured.
- **Medication:** The usual medications which are administered to the patient in diarrhea are antidiarrheal, demulcents, astringents, antiseptics, sedatives and antispasmodic should be given.

CARE OF DYSPNEA PATIENT

- **Psychological support:** A dyspneic patient is very anxious and he needs to be reassured. The nurse in the care of the patient should stand with the patient and encourage him.
- **Ventilation of the room:** The room should be well-ventilated to supply fresh air to the patient avoid overcrowding.
- **Ventilation of lungs:** If the respiratory mechanism is falling, the ventilation of the lungs can be achieved by artificial respiration.
- **Positioning of the patient:** The most appropriate position for a dyspneic patient is a propped up position which can be maintained by the backrest and extra pillows.
- **Oxygen inhalation:** If the patient is cyanosed it indicates the lack of oxygen supply in the tissue. Oxygen is given.

- **Clearance of the air passage:** It has to be cleared by appropriate means, e.g. by the use of mechanical suction.
- **Breathing and coughing exercise:** The patient is asked to cough and the sputum.
- **Postural drainage:** If there is secretions collected in the lungs, postural drainage will help to drain the secretions.
- **Steam inhalation:** The steam inhalations facilitates to smoothen the mucosa and to liquefy the sputum.
- **Nutrition:** Small and frequent diet offers to patient. Avoid overloading of stomach to prevent dyspnea.

6. Write short notes on any four of the following:

(a) Snake bite
(b) Records and reports
(c) Heat transmission
(d) O_2 administration
(e) Importance of first aid

SNAKE BITE

All snakes are not poisonous. The snake must be identified because not antivenin is necessary if it is nonpoisonous. If the snake cannot be identified it should be treated as poisonous, and general antivenin should be given.

First Aid Measures for Snake Bites are:

- Lay the patient down and reassure him.
- Apply a broad firm bandage above the bitten area. It should allow entry of a finger do not lessen it periodically like a tourniquet.
- Immobilize the bitten limb with splints to reduce lymphatic flow and spread of the poison.
- Leave bandage and splint in position till medical care is available.
- Wash bitten area with plain water or soap and water.
- Arrange for immediate transfer to a hospital.
- Give first aid for unconsciousness respiratory arrest or cardiac arrest.
- If bite is at a place where crave bandage cannot be applied, then:
  - Wash bitten area
  - Make a 3 mm deep cut through each fang marks with sterile razor, blade to facilitate bleeding and drainage of venous
  - Apply ice-pack locally
  - Keep patient still
  - Arrange for transfer to hospital.

- Cauterization of wound and applications of potassium permanganate crystals locally is controversial.

RECORDS AND REPORTS

The patient's clinical record is a brief account of the personal and medical history of the patient, results of diagnostic test, findings of medical examination, treatment and nursing care, daily progress notes and advice on discharge.

Records

Health records refer to forms on which information about an individual and family is noted.

Principles of Records

- Records must be written clearly
- Records are legal documents and should contain true facts based on observation conversation and action
- Records should be briefly and clearly noted
- It should have accurate and complete information
- Records should be written immediately after event
- It should be neat and clean
- Not handover to any strange person.

Uses of Records

- Effective in communication
- Helps in providing best possible services to individual and community
- Can save effort and money
- Health worker can organize his work
- Useful in research
- Useful in health education.

Values of Records

- Records provide an accurate and detailed account of treatment and care given
- It provides information of the result of medication and treatment given to the patient
- There are of great help in diagnosis, treatment and nursing care
- It prevents duplication of work in future
- It has legal valve

- It is helpful for medical students
- They provide reference material for research work
- They provide information about the health problems of the country.

Reports

Reports are effective method of communication among the members of the health team. Reports provide information about patient either written or oral.

Purposes

- To show the kind and amount of service rendered over a special period
- To illustrate progress in reaching goals
- Aids in studying health conditions and planning
- To interpret the services to the public and to the other interested agencies.

Care of Records and Reports

- All records and reports are kept under the safe custody of nurse in each ward or department
- No individual sheet is separated from the complete records
- Records are kept in a place, not permitted to patient and visitors
- Records are not handed over to the legal advisors without the written permission of the administrator
- All records are to be handled carefully, careless handling can destroy records
- All records are filled according to the hospital custom
- Records are never sent out of the hospital without the doctor's permission.

HEAT TRANSMISSION

Heat is transferred from the warmer to the cooler region. Heat is transferred by these methods.

1. Conduction
2. Convection
3. Radiation

Conduction

It is the transfer of heat directly through a substance from hot part to cold part, from one molecule to the other. Heat is transferred by conduction from the body to any substance in contract with the body such as air, clothes, food stuffs, water, etc. Very little heat is lost by conduction.

Convection

It is the method of the transfer of heat by circulating air or liquid and it depends open the our movement and the temperature of the atmosphere.

Radiation

Radiation is the transfer of heat from the surface of one object to that on another which is not in contact with one another. These waves travel through the space without causing any appreciable change in the temperature of the air about 60% of the body heat is lost by radiation.

Application of Heat Transfer in the Body

- Heat energy produced in the body from oxidation of food stuffs in the tissues.
- Heat energy lost from body by conduction and radiation. Normally, the body looses about 100 calories/Hour.
- Most of the heat of body is lost through the skin.
- A hot bath transfers heat to the body and increases metabolism bathing in a cold water causes loss of heat from skin.
- Heat is lost by evaporation of perspiration by expired air, by blood supply in lungs, by urination and defecation.

O_2 ADMINISTRATION

Patient with respiratory dysfunctions are treated with oxygen inhalation

Indications

- Cyanosis
- Breathlessness
- Environment low in oxygen
- Dyspnea
- Anemia
- Disease of lungs

- Poisoning and chemicals
- Shock and circulatory failure
- Hemorrhage and air hunger
- Patient under anesthesia
- Asphyxia
- Patient who are critically ill.

Methods of Oxygen Administration

- Oxygen by nasal catheter
- Oxygen by mask
- Oxygen tent.

Precautions

The following precautions should be taken:

- The proper O_2 cylinder or pipeline
- No blockage in the catheter or no leakage to be present
- Humidified O_2 should be given to avoid burning of mucous membrane
- Give intermittent O_2 and not the continuous and as advised by doctor
- Check the improvement in patient condition after O_2 inhalation
- Do not use flaming items as match box, rubber toys or do not smoke at that area
- Check the apparatus daily in order to meet in an emergency or its functioning conditions.

Hazards of O_2 Inhalation

- Infection
- Combustion
- Oxygen toxicity
- Atelectasis
- Oxygen induced apnea
- Retrolental fibroplasia
- Asphyxia.

IMPORTANCE OF FIRST AID

- To preserve life
- To relieve pain
- To prevent further injury and deterioration of the condition of the patient
- To make medical care available at the earliest.

Fundamental of Nursing
September 2005

Time: 3 Hours **Maximum Marks: 75**

Note: *Attempt all questions. Attempt all parts of the questions in continuity.*

1. **Define the following:** **1×10=10**
   (a) Nursing
   (b) Antiseptic
   (c) Cyanosis
   (d) Surface tension
   (e) Isolation
   (f) Diffusion
   (g) Friction
   (h) Hemoptysis
   (i) Temperature
   (j) Rigor mortis
2. **Enlist the Following:** **2×5=10**
   (a) Purposes of soap and water enema.
   (b) Purposes of mouth care.
   (c) Purposes of Fowler's position.
   (d) Precautions while collecting urine specimen.
3. **(a) Write down the nursing principles used in nursing procedures.** **5+5+5=15**
   (b) Write in detail the procedure of taking blood pressure.
   (c) Write the procedure of steam inhalation.
4. **(a) Write down the functions of a nurse.** **5+5=10**
   (b) Define comfort devices and its uses.
5. **(a) Define hyperpyrexia.** **2+3+5=10**
   (b) Write the stages of rigor.
   (c) What nursing measures will you take for a patient having fever?
6. **Write short notes on any four of the following:** **5×4=20**
   (a) Golden rules of first aid
   (b) Shock
   (c) Types of levers
   (d) Functions of hospital
   (e) Cold compresses

SOLVED QUESTION PAPER 2005

1. Define the following:

(a) Nursing
(b) Antiseptic
(c) Cyanosis
(d) Surface tension
(e) Isolation
(f) Diffusion
(g) Friction
(h) Hemoptysis
(i) Temperature
(j) Rigor mortis

NURSING

According to INC

Nursing is the unique function of a nurse that is to assist the individual side or well in the performance of those activities contributing to health or its recovery that he would perform unaided if he had the necessary strength, will or knowledge.

ANTISEPTIC

It is process of sterilization use chemical substance to prevent the infection or the growth of the organism is known as antiseptic.

CYANOSIS

It is blueness or discoloration of the skin and mucous membrance due to lack of oxygen in the body tissue.

SURFACE TENSION

It is the tendency of the surface of liquid to minimise the area of its surface by contracting.

ISOLATION

It is the separation of infected person to healthy person to prevent the spreading of communicable disease.

DIFFUSION

It is the spontaneous mixing of molecules of liquid or gas to that they become equally distributed.

FRICTION

It is act of rubbing when one object surface moves across another frictional forces oppose that motion.

HEMOPTYSIS

Coughing out of blood with sputum is known as hemoptysis, e.g. in tuberculosis.

TEMPERATURE

It is the balance between heat lost and heat gained by the body.

RIGOR MORTIS

It is the stiffening of the body after death within few hours because of coagulation of muscle plasma.

2. Enlist the following:

(a) Purposes of soap and water enema
(b) Purposes of mouth care
(c) Purposes of Fowler's position
(d) Precautions while collecting urine specimen

PURPOSES OF SOAP AND WATER ENEMA

- To relieve constipation
- To use before bowel wash
- Use before delivery
- Before major surgery done under general anesthesia
- Before barium enema
- To relieve gases.

PURPOSES OF MOUTH CARE

- To clean the mouth
- To feel fresh and to increase appetite
- To increase the blood circulation
- To prevent dental caries and systemic infection
- To make the gums healthy
- To prevent from oral infection
- To provide clean appearance to mouth and face.

PURPOSES OF FOWLER'S POSITION

- To relive dyspnea
- After abdominal surgery on 2nd or 3rd day
- To give one of the positions to a very sick patient e.g. asthmatic patient
- To serve a diet to patient.

PRECAUTIONS WHILE COLLECTING URINE SPECIMEN

Ask patients to clean the genital area with soap and water and then rinse with water alone. In female patient, the labia are separated for cleaning and kept apart until the urine has been collected. In male patient, the foreskin should be retracted and the glans penis is cleaned before the collection of the urine.

- Give clean bedpan to the patient who not able to go for bathroom
- Use sterile container for collection of urine
- Prevent the container from soiling outside
- Close the container when collect the specimen
- Label the container by necessary information like name, age, and sex and bed no., ward no. of patient
- Send the specimen in laboratory for investigation.

3. (a) Write down the nursing principles used in nursing procedures.

(b) Write in detail the procedure of taking blood pressure.

(c) Write the procedure of steam inhalation.

NURSING PRINCIPLES USED IN NURSING PROCEDURES

- ***Safety:*** It means prevention of mechanical, thermal, chemical and bacteriological injuries to the patient and protect from all injuries.
- ***Therapeutic effectiveness:*** It means to achieve the purpose for which a procedure is done.
- ***Comfort:*** To provide comfort to the patient and the worker by using veterinary specialist group task, e.g. change the position of patient and give rest to staff after completing duty hours.
- ***Use of resources:*** It includes used of time, money and material in effective manner.
- ***Good workmanship:*** It is art of doing work with skill and knowledge with the safety of patient.
- ***Individuality:*** Provide care to another individual patient against particular event. Do the procedure according to need of patient without harm of patient.

TAKING OF BLOOD PRESSURE PROCEDURE

- Explain the procedure to patient.
- While taking BP, the patient should be relaxed.
- Give comfortable position to patient preferred lying position.
- Bring all the articles near to bedside and provide privacy. Ask the patient for bedpan and urinal for a bedridden patient, so that patient should not ask it during the procedure.
- The cuff on right hand or left hand above the elbow joint tightly.
- The apparatus should be kept parallel to heart not low or high to get correct reading.
- Pump the cuff till mercury reached to the 200 point
- Put stethoscope on the cubital fossa to hear the sound of artery and gradually unlock the screw to get the sound.
- A sound listen when unlock the screw first systolic and second sound is diastolic.
- Record the BP in unit of mm Hg.
- Record the BP range if it high or low informs to sister incharge.
- If you are unable to get proper readings ask to sister incharge for help.
- One hand the BP should not be checked more than three times.
- Loose the cuff and remove.
- Make the patient comfortable.
- Record the BP on patient chart with date and time.

STEAM INHALATION PROCEDURE

- Select the patient to whom the steam has to be given.
- Explain the procedure to patient to make a patient comfortable.
- Prepare the patient physically and mentally.
- Give comfortable position to patient and offer bedpan and urinal as required.
- Use Fowler's position with cardiac table if patient is able to sit.
- In bedridden patient the side lying position can be given.
- Put off all fan, close doors and windows.
- Arrange all articles near bedside.
- Prepared inhaler should be gives to the patient by putting free spout on the opposite side of the patient.
- Cover the patient with inhaler except spout outside.
- Instruct the patient to inhale the steam by putting the lips on the mouth piece and exhales through nose.
- It has to be continued for 15 to 20 minutes.

- Keep sputum mug within reach of patient to the sputum.
- Do not leave the patient alone.
- Do not permit to go out and switch on the fan.
- Wipe the sweat from the face.
- Assess the patient for effectiveness of the procedure.
- Terminate the procedure.
- Record the detail of procedure.
- Give comfortable position.
- Replace all the articles.

4. (a) Write down the functions of a nurse.
(b) Define comfort devices and its uses.

FUNCTIONS OF A NURSE

A professional nurse has the following functions:

- To provide basic nursing care her patients.
- To administer to medications and treatment prescribed by the physician.
- To observe patients response and adaptation to illness.
- To observe patients response and adaptation to treatments.
- To teach self-care and counsel on health matters.
- To supervise or guide the patient in rehabilitative activities related to daily living.
- To participate in research works related to health care.
- To plan with the patient in such a manner as to develop a sense of trust self worth.
- To plan and teach the patient and his family relation to the restoration and promotion of health and prevention of disease.
- To coordinate the services of all groups contributing to the care of the patient, his family and society.
- To teach and supervise the nursing students and other auxiliary personal.
- To maintain her own physical and mental health.

COMFORT DEVICE AND ITS USES

Define

Comfort devices are those devices which are used for the comfort of patient in various conditions, some use for positioning, some for prevent pressure on body parts. These are the following:

- ***Backrest:*** It is a mechanical device which provides support for the patient in the sitting position.

- ***Knee rest:*** Knee rest may be substituted by a pillow, give relaxation and relieve pain on abdominal muscles and on tendon beneath the knees.
- ***Footrest:*** It helps to maintain the normal position of the feet, i.e. at right angles to the leg. It is used for the comfort and to prevent foot drop. Hard pillows, sand bags or foot board, etc. are substituted for this.
- ***Bed cradle:*** It used to support and take off the weight of the top bed clothing, prevent the top cloth coming in contact the patient as in case of patients with burns.
- ***Bed blocks:*** Bed blocks are made-up of wood or metal and used to raise the foot end or head and of the bed. Bed block are used to prevent shock, to arrest hemorrhage, to retain enema and after giving spinal anesthesia.
- ***Sand bags:*** Sand bags are used to immobilize a part as in fractures and to relieve discomfort. It may also be used to give support in any part of the body and to prevent food drop or wrist drop.
- ***Air cushion:*** Air cushion is made-up of rubber and it can be inflated with air. It is used to relieve pressure on certain parts of the body.
- ***Rubber and cotton rings:*** It is used to relieve pressure on certain parts of the body like elbow and heels.
- ***Air and water mattress:*** These are used for very thin and very obese patients and those who are prone to pressure sores. Pressure exerted by body will be distributed equally in all directions and prevent to development of pressure sores.

5. (a) Define hyperpyrexia.

(b) Write the stages of rigor.

(c) What nursing measures will you take for a patient having fever?

HYPERPYREXIA

The temperature goes above 105°C is called hyperpyrexia.

STAGES OF RIGOR

Rigor is characterised by three stages:

- **The first stage or cold stage:** The patient shivers uncontrollably. The skin is cold, face is pinched and pale, the pulse is feeble and rapid. The temperature rises rapidly to 103°F or above. In this stage, cover the patient with blankets and apply warmth give warm drinks. Protect the patient from falling.
- **The second stage or hot stage:** The skin feels hot and dry and patient feels very thirsty. The shivering stops. The patient may restless. The temperature may continue to rise.

During 2nd stage, remove all blankets and hot applications. Give him cool drinks. Cold compress apply to relieve congestion and headache. If temperature congestion and headache goes to very high above 105°F cold sponging may be start and record temperature every 10 to 15 minutes.

- **Third stage or stage of sweating:** The patient sweats profusely TP falls. The pulse improve patient feel some comfort. During this stage, change clothes of patient give sponge and dry the patient. Continuous watching of TPR at every 15 minutes necessary without disturbing the patient.

NURSING CARE IN FEVER REGULATION OF BODY TEMPERATURE

Case of the patients in fevers focuses on reducing the elevated body temperature, when a patient's temperature is high various method used for cooling the body are:

- Exposure to cool air by an electric fan
- Administration of cool drinks
- Application of cold compress and ice bags
- Cold sponging and cold packs
- Cold bath
- Ice cold lavages and enemas
- Use of hypothermic blankets or mattresses.

But care should be taken during use of these method, to prevent of occurring of shivering:

- **Meeting the nutritional need:** The cellular metabolism is greatly increased during fever and increase oxygen consumption 13% for each °C and 7% for each therefore, a high caloric diet is indicated in fevers. Most of the patients refer fluid diet. The fluid intake is increased to 3000 mL in 24 hours to prevent dehydration and to eliminate the waste products:
  - If nausea, vomiting present IV fluid given with the permission of physician.
  - If there is burning micturition encourage the patient to take plenty of water (fluid).
  - Intake output chart maintained.
  - The patient who tolerate solid diet should be given attractive food to increase the appetite according to like and dislike of patient.
  - A diet which is soft and containing plenty of fluids and fruits will help to evacuate the bowel regularly.
- **Providing rest and sleep:** Provide proper rest and sleep to all patients who are suffering from fever. Provide proper unit free from noise, glaze

of light and comfortable bed, change position frequently to prevent pressure sore.

- **Maintenance of personal Hygiene:**
  - **Mouth care:** Mouth care very essential for patient who is having fever from many days. It oral hygiene is not maintained various problem, arise, e.g. coated tongue, parotitis, crusts, etc. provide frequently mouth care is essential.
  - **Skin care:** Care of skin is essential to prevent bedsores. Sponge both is given daily to keep a patient clean is and change clothes daily. Special attention is given to pressure points.
- **Safety factors:** Never leave the patient alone with high grade fever. If fever over 103°F for a long time it may lead to delirium and convulsion. Prevent the patient from fall down. If the temperature is not coming down with cold sponging. Antipyretic drugs, e.g. paracetamol may be given with advise of the doctor.
- **Observation of patient:** Patient requires frequent and intelligence observation by the nurses. The vital signs are to be checked frequently to know the regression and progress of the disease. When any type of cold application are applied. The temperature taken by rectum to get accurate temperature maintain TPR chart of patient.

6. Write short notes on any four of the following:

(a) Golden rules of first aid
(b) Shock
(c) Types of lever
(d) Functions of hospital
(e) Cold compresses

GOLDEN RULES OF FIRST AID

- Reach the site of accident as early as possible.
- Do not waste time asking unnecessary questions.
- Find old the cause of the injury.
- Separate the causative agent from the patient or the patient from the agent, e.g. falling machinery, fire, electrical/line wire, poisonous insects, etc.
- Find out whether the patient is dead or alive, conscious or unconscious.
- Determine the priority of first aid measures to be adopted, e.g. restoration of cardiac function, restoration of breathing, stop bleeding from the site of injury, etc. in the order.
- Arrange for medical aid.

- Keep a record of the patient and the details of the event.
- Keep the patient warm and comfortable as far as possible.
- Improvise rather than wait for specific equipment.
- If the patient is conscious, reassure him.

SHOCK

- Immediately reassure and comfort the casualty.
- Provide position to relieving shock.
- Lower extremities should be elevated.
- Keep the patient warm and cover with a blanket.
- Loose tight clothes to help the circulation and assist breathing.
- Find out cause of shock and treat it.
- If shock occurs due to bleeding, stop the bleeding.
- Check for fracture and immobilize fracture.
- Check breathing rate, pulse and level of consciousness.
- It breathing and heart beat stop, then establish an airway and start resuscitation immediately.
- Keep the patient in recovery position.
- Shift patient to hospital immediately.

TYPES OF LEVER

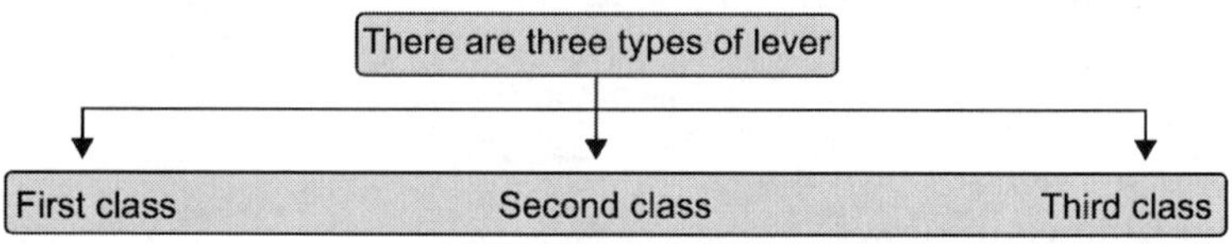

- ***First class lever:*** The fulcrum is in the middle the load is at one end and the effort is at the other, e.g. pressing of pedal.
- ***Second class lever:*** The fulcrum is at one end, the load is in middle and the effort is at the other, e.g. turning firm mattress.
- ***Third class lever:*** The fulcrum is at one end, the load is at the other end and effort is in the middle, e.g. using of forceps.

FUNCTIONS OF HOSPITAL

- **Care of the sick and injured:** Hospital is an institute where care is provide to sick and injured person by trained and skill staff.
- **Prevention of disease and promotion of health:** In hospital, medical staff provides service to prevent from disease and promotion of health of people.

- **Diagnosis and treatment of disease:** Hospital services help to find out the diagnosis of disease and in providing best possible treatment of disease.
- **Medical education:** Hospitals are helpful for the student's education who attached with medical profession.
- **Research:** Hospital records helpful in research activities because hospital serve useful data.
- **Immunization:** Immunization against six killer diseases is done in every hospital and also against other disease.
- **Rehabilitation:** Rehabilitation services provided in hospital to disabled or patient who recover from chronic sickness.

COLD COMPRESSES

This is a local moist cold application made out of folded layers of gauze, lint piece or old soft linen wring out of cold or ice water and applied to the required area, it is left uncovered.

Purposes

- To reduce swelling
- To reduce pain
- To control pain
- To decrease/reduce pyrexia
- To check the growth of bacteria
- To control hemorrhage.